安徽省教育厅高等学校省级质量工程一流教材建设项目
（2021yljc066）
医学英语新医科课程群系列教材

医学英语综合教程

Medical English: An Integrated Course

（第4次修订）

主　编　汪　媛　庞　炜

副主编　王　然　李雪梅　徐　燕

编　者　（按姓氏笔画为序）

王　然　王栩彬　王燕茹

刘　军　刘娅敏　刘维静

李洪伟　李雪梅　杨红梅

汪　媛　张自云　庞　炜

徐　燕　曹凤隆　蔡　郁

U0250615

南京大学出版社

图书在版编目(CIP)数据

医学英语综合教程 / 汪媛，庞炜主编. — 南京：
南京大学出版社，2023.12
ISBN 978 - 7 - 305 - 26977 - 6

Ⅰ. ①医… Ⅱ. ①汪… ②庞… Ⅲ. ①医学－英语－
高等学校－教材 Ⅳ. ①R

中国国家版本馆 CIP 数据核字(2023)第 090170 号

出版发行　南京大学出版社
社　　址　南京市汉口路 22 号　　　　邮　编　210093
书　　名　医学英语综合教程
　　　　　　YIXUE YINGYU ZONGHE JIAOCHENG
主　　编　汪　媛　庞　炜
责任编辑　裴维维　　　　　　　　　编辑热线　025 - 83592123
照　　排　南京南琳图文制作有限公司
印　　刷　盐城市华光印刷厂
开　　本　787 mm×1092 mm　1/16　印张 11.5　字数 360 千
版　　次　2023 年 12 月第 1 版　2023 年 12 月第 1 次印刷
ISBN 978 - 7 - 305 - 26977 - 6
定　　价　47.00 元

网址：http://www.njupco.com
官方微博：http://weibo.com/njupco
官方微信号：njupress
销售咨询热线：(025) 83594756

前　言

　　医学生的培养质量关乎人民健康,高质量的医学人才是推进国家卫生健康事业发展的重要基础和有力保障。当前,人民日益增长的健康需求和全面推进健康中国建设对医学教育提出了更高要求。2018年以来颁布的《关于加快建设高水平本科教育 全面提高人才培养能力的意见》《关于加强医教协同实施卓越医生教育培养计划2.0的意见》《关于实施基础学科拔尖学生培养计划2.0的意见》《高等学校课程思政建设指导纲要》《大学英语教学指南》《关于加快医学教育创新发展的指导意见》等一系列教育指导性文件为高校医学人才的培养提供了目标方向和实施指导意见。

　　为顺应时代发展,遵循国家和社会对培养新时代"五术"医学人才的要求,我们在十余年医学英语教学实践和教学改革成果基础之上,对《医学英语综合教程》(第三版)进行了全面改版,立足以学生为中心的教育理念,完善教材设计,使之更好地满足国家、社会和个人学习的需求。

一、教材特色

特色1:"外语+医学"的医文融合特点

　　本教材为通用英语与双语或全英文专业医学英语课程之间的桥梁课程所用教材,将医学专业基础课程内容与语言学习相融合,各单元以解剖学、生理学、生物化学等医学专业基础与临床课程为主题,单元内容与医学生专业知识架构贴合,利于学生未来深入学习高阶专业英语课程或开展自学。

特色2:课程思政教学元素

　　人文精神是医学的核心价值,现代医学已由传统的生物医学模式向生物—心理—社会医学模式转变,患者需要有温度的医学,医生更要在解除患者病痛时自觉践行人文关怀,给予患者精神慰藉。教材通过医学人文热点话题的篇章阅读和口语展示或讨论鼓励学生追寻医学史和医学人物,辩证分析思考当代医学热点,加深对"医者乃生死所寄,责任重大,非仁爱之士,不可托也"的理解,为自觉弘扬"敬佑生命、救死扶伤、甘于奉献、大爱无疆"的职业精神奠定认知基础。

特色3:多技能语言综合训练

　　本教材的练习设计注重听、说、读、写、译相互融合的多技能训练,如每单元Oral

Presentation and Discussion 部分的练习设计为读后陈述和观后讨论,将阅读与口语训练、自主学习慕课与口头讨论相结合,语言单技能训练之间有机转换,有效提升学生语言综合应用和跨文化交际能力。再如,每个单元的写作练习为单元中快速阅读材料的主旨概要写作,学生可以医学主题文章为范本,通过阅读了解医学语篇的写作特点,并进行模仿,完成语言输入—语言输出的转换,提高写作能力与学习效能。

特色 4:配套线上课程开发

基于多年的教学实践,我们已开发完成与教材配套的慕课,目前已上线国家级慕课教学平台学堂在线,相关慕课内容可作为纸质教材内容和线下教学的补充,也可供教师以线上线下混合式教学模式开展教学。

二、修订内容说明

本教材此次改版修订主要体现在以下方面:

删减内容:将原有 16 个单元删减压缩至 10 个单元,从而更好地适应当前课堂学时缩减的现状。

替换内容:替换 7 个单元中 Oral Presentation and Discussion 部分已失去时效的阅读文本,代之以医学人文热点为主题的文本;替换 5 个单元与单元主题不相符的主课文和快速阅读篇章;替换每单元中医学英语摘要写作与翻译部分过于陈旧的语言例证;重新编写替换每个单元的听力部分。

补充内容:增加每单元医学术语以及翻译写作版块的练习比重与练习形式,通过匹配题、填空题、改错题以及英汉互译等练习类型,凸显学练结合、以学生为中心的教学理念。

《医学英语综合教程》第一版于 2010 年编写出版,之后的 10 余年间在原有教学实践基础之上历经两次改版,内容不断更新完善。本教材曾入选安徽省普通高等教育"十一五"规划教材与"十二五"规划教材,本次教材的改版修订再次获得安徽省教育厅高等学校省级质量工程一流教材建设项目立项。但因书号系统调整,本教材版次未能沿用。

本教材于 2010 年编写之初,丁启鹏、朱同生两位教授审看本书并提出宝贵建议,教材历次使用与改版修订均得到了安徽医科大学外语系全体教师的大力支持和建言献策,本次改版修订也得到原一至三版教材主编蔡郁教授的倾力指导,在此一并致谢。

由于编者水平有限,书中难免存在疏漏和不足,敬请同行专家和教材使用者批评指正。

编　者
2023 年 12 月

Contents

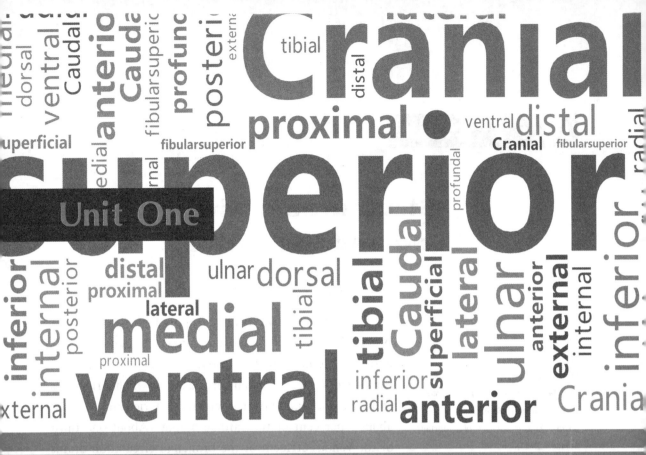

Unit One

Anatomy

✓课文音频
✓听力音频
✓在线课程
✓课件申请

Structures of the Lung and the Kidney

The Blood Vessels of the Lung

vascular /ˈvæskjələ/ adj. 血管的，脉管的

bronchial /ˈbrɒŋkiəl/ adj. 支气管的

alveolar /ælˈviːələ/ adj. （alveolus n., pl. alveoli）肺泡的

aorta /eɪˈɔːtə/ n. （pl. aortae/ aortas）主动脉

intercostal /ˌɪntə(ː)ˈkɒstl/ adj. 肋间的

ventricle /ˈventrɪkl/ n. （脑、心）室

thebesian /θiːˈbiːziən/ veins 心最小静脉（特贝西乌斯静脉）

shunt /ʃʌnt/ n. 分流管

periphery /pəˈrɪfəri/ n. 外周，周围

arteriole /ɑːˈtɪəriəʊl/ n. 小动脉

capillary /kəˈpɪləri/ n. 毛细血管

hilum /ˈhaɪləm/ n. （pl. hila）门

atrium /ˈeɪtriəm/ n. 心房

The lung receives its blood supply from two vascular systems—the bronchial and pulmonary circulations. The nutritive blood flow to all but the alveolar structures comes from the bronchial circulation, which originates from the aorta and upper intercostal arteries and receives about 1 per cent of the cardiac output. About one third of the venous effluent of the bronchial circulation drains into the systemic veins and back to the right ventricle. The remainder drains into the pulmonary veins and, along with the contribution from the thebesian veins in the heart, represents a component of the 1 to 2 per cent right-to-left shunt found in normal subjects.

The pulmonary arterial system runs alongside the airways from the hila to the periphery. The arteries down to the level of the subsegmental airways (2 mm diameter) are thin-walled, predominantly elastic vessels. Beyond this, the arteries become muscularized until they reach diameters of 30 μm, at which point the muscular coat disappears. Most of the arterial pressure drop takes place in these small muscular arteries, which are responsible for the active control of blood flow distribution in the lung. The pulmonary arterioles empty into an extensive capillary network and drain into thin-walled pulmonary veins, which eventually join with the arteries and bronchi at the hilum and exit the lung to enter the left atrium.

Elements of Renal Structure

The human kidneys are anatomically positioned in the retroperitoneal space at level of the lower thoracic and upper lumbar vertebrae. Each adult kidney weighs approximately 150 g and measures about 12 by 6 by 3 cm. A coronal section of the kidney reveals two distinct regions. The outer region, the cortex, is about 1 cm in thickness. The inner region is the medulla and is made up of several conical structures. The bases of these pyramidal structures are located at the corticomedullary junction, and the apices extend into the hilum of the kidney as the papillae. Each papilla is enclosed by a minor calyx; these calyces collectively communicate with major calyces, forming the renal pelvis. Urine that flows from the papillae is collected in the renal pelvis and passes to the bladder through the ureters.

Blood is delivered to each kidney from a main renal artery branching from the aorta. The main artery usually divides into two main segmental branches, which are further subdivided into lobar arteries supplying the upper, middle, and lower regions of the kidney. These vessels subdivide further as they enter the renal parenchyma and create interlobar arteries that course toward the renal cortex. These smaller arteries provide perpendicular branches, the arcuate arteries, at the corticomedullary junction. Interlobular arteries arising from the arcuates extend into the cortex. The glomerular capillaries receive blood through afferent arterioles that originate from these terminal interlobular arteries.

Histologically, the kidney is composed of a basic structural unit known as the nephron. Each human kidney contains approximately 1 million nephrons. The nephron is composed of two major components: a filtering element composed of an enclosed capillary network (the glomerulus) and an attached tubule. The tubule contains several distinct anatomic and functional segments.

retroperitoneal /ˌretrəʊˌperɪtəˈnɪəl/ space 腹膜后隙

thoracic /θɔːˈræsɪk/ adj. 胸的，胸廓的

vertebra /ˈvɜːtɪbrə/ n. 脊椎骨，椎骨

coronal /ˈkɒrənl/ adj. 冠状的

cortex /ˈkɔːteks/ n. (pl. cortices /ˈkɔːtɪsiːz/ or cortexes) 皮质

medulla /meˈdʌlə/ n. (pl. medullas or medullae /meˈdʌliː/) 髓质

corticomedullary junction 皮髓质结合

apex /ˈeɪpeks/ n. (pl. apices /ˈeɪpɪˌsiːz/) 顶尖

papilla /pəˈpɪlə/ n. (pl. papillae /pəˈpɪliː/) 乳突

calyx /ˈkeɪlɪks/ n. (pl. calyces) 盏

renal /ˈriːnl/ adj. 肾的

renal pelvis /ˈpelvɪs/ 肾盂

ureter /jʊəˈriːtə/ n. 输尿管

parenchyma /pəˈreŋkɪmə/ n. 实质

arcuate /ˈɑːkjʊɪt/ artery /ˈɑːtəri/ 弓状动脉

glomerular /ɡlɒˈmeruːlə/ adj. 肾小球的

afferent /ˈæfərənt/ adj. 传入的

nephron /ˈnefrɒn/ n. 肾单位

glomerulus /ɡlɒˈmeruːləs/ n. (pl. glomeruli /ɡlɒˈmeruːlaɪ/) (肾)小球

Task 1 Find out the answers to the following questions and then compare your answers with a partner.

1. Where do the lungs get their blood supply?

2. Does the nutritive blood flow to the alveolar structures?

3. What is/are responsible for the active control of blood flow distribution in the lung?

4. Where do afferent arterioles come from?

5. What do the interlobular arteries provide at the corticomedullary junction?

Part Ⅱ Listening

Task 2 You will hear 20 words or phrases which will be read three times. Write them down on the blanks and check with your partner after you finish.

1. _____   2. _____   3. _____   4. _____

5. _____   6. _____   7. _____   8. _____

9. _____   10. _____   11. _____   12. _____

13. _____   14. _____   15. _____   16. _____

17. _____   18. _____   19. _____   20. _____

Task 3 You are going to hear a passage which will be read three times. Take some notes while you are listening to the passage and then answer the following questions.

1. What is anatomical position?

_____

2. Why is anatomical position important?

_____

3. When may the terms "prone" and "supine" be used?

_____

Part III Oral Presentation and Discussion

 Task 4 **Read the following passage and make an oral presentation.**

Coronary Artery Disease

What Is Coronary Artery Disease?

Coronary artery disease occurs when fatty deposits called plaque (say "plak") build up inside the coronary arteries. The coronary arteries wrap around the heart and supply it with blood and oxygen. When plaque builds up, it narrows the arteries and reduces the amount of blood that gets to your heart. This can lead to serious problems, including heart attack.

Coronary artery disease (also called CAD) is the most common type of heart disease. It is also the number one killer of both men and women in the United States.

It can be a shock to find out that you have coronary artery disease. Many people only find out when they have a heart attack. Whether or not you have had a heart attack, there are many things you can do to slow coronary artery disease and reduce your risk of future problems.

What Causes Coronary Artery Disease?

Coronary artery disease is caused by hardening of the arteries, or atherosclerosis. Atherosclerosis occurs when plaque builds up inside the arteries. (Arteries are the blood vessels that carry oxygen-rich blood throughout your body.) Atherosclerosis can affect any arteries in the body. When it occurs in the arteries that supply blood to the heart, it is called coronary artery disease.

Plaque is a fatty material made up of cholesterol, calcium, and other substances in the blood. To understand why plaque is a problem, compare a healthy artery with an artery with atherosclerosis:

- A healthy artery is like a rubber tube. It is smooth and flexible, and blood flows through it freely. If your heart has to work harder, such as when you exercise, a healthy artery can stretch to let more blood flow to your body's tissues.
- An artery with atherosclerosis is more like a clogged pipe. Plaque narrows the artery and makes it stiff. This limits the flow of blood to the tissues. When the heart has to work harder, the stiff arteries can't flex to let more blood through, and the tissues don't get enough blood and oxygen.

When plaque builds up in the coronary arteries, the heart doesn't get the blood it needs to work well. Over time, this can weaken or damage the heart. If a plaque tears, the body tries to fix the tear by forming a blood clot around it. The clot can block blood flow to the heart and cause a heart attack.

What Are the Symptoms?

Usually people with coronary artery disease don't have symptoms until after age 50. Then they may start to have symptoms at times when the heart is working harder and needs more oxygen, such as during exercise. Typical first symptoms include:

- Chest pain, called angina.
- Shortness of breath.
- Heart attack. Too often, a heart attack is the first symptom of coronary artery disease.

Some people don't have symptoms. In rare cases, a person can have a "silent" heart attack, without symptoms.

How Is Coronary Artery Disease Diagnosed?

To diagnose coronary artery disease, doctors start by doing a physical exam and asking questions about your past health and your risk factors. Risk factors are things that increase the chance that you will have coronary artery disease.

Some common risk factors are being older than 65; smoking; having high cholesterol, high blood pressure, or diabetes; and having heart disease in your family. The more risk factors you have, the more likely it is that you have coronary artery disease.

If your doctor thinks you have coronary artery disease, you may have tests, such as:

- Electrocardiogram (EKG or ECG), which checks for problems with the electrical activity of your heart.
- Chest X-ray.
- Blood tests.
- Exercise electrocardiogram, commonly called a "stress test". This test checks for changes in your heart while you exercise.

Your doctor may order other tests to look at blood flow to your heart. You may have a coronary angiogram if your doctor is considering a procedure to remove blockages, such as angioplasty or bypass surgery.

How Is It Treated?

Treatment focuses on taking steps to manage your symptoms and reduce your risk for heart attack and stroke. Some risk factors you can't control, such as your age or family history. Other risks you can control, such as high blood pressure and high cholesterol. Lifestyle changes can help lower your risks. You may also need to take medicines or have a procedure to open your arteries.

Lifestyle changes are the first step for anyone with coronary artery disease. These changes may stop or even reverse coronary artery disease. To improve your heart health:

- Don't smoke. This may be the most important thing you can do. Quitting smoking can quickly reduce the risk of heart attack or death.
- Eat a heart-healthy diet that includes plenty of fish, fruits, vegetables, beans, high-fiber grains and breads, and olive oil. This is sometimes called a Mediterranean diet. See a dietitian if you need help making better food choices.
- Get regular exercise on most, preferably all, days of the week. Your doctor can suggest a safe level of exercise for you. Walking is great exercise that most people can do.
- Lower your stress level. Stress can damage your heart.

Changing old habits may not be easy, but it is very important to help you live a healthier and longer life. Having a plan can help.

Start with small steps. For example, commit to eating five servings of fruits and vegetables a day. Instead of having dessert, take a short walk. When you feel stressed, stop and take some deep breaths.

Procedures may be done to improve blood flow to the heart.

- Angioplasty is the treatment doctors prefer, because it isn't major surgery. During angioplasty, the doctor guides a thin tube (catheter) into the narrowed artery and inflates a small balloon. This widens the artery to help restore blood flow. Often a small wire-mesh tube called a stent is placed to keep the artery open. The doctor may use a stent that is coated with medicine, called a drug-eluting stent. When the stent is in place, it slowly releases a medicine that prevents the growth of new tissue. This helps keep the artery open.

- Bypass surgery may be a better choice in some cases, such as if more than one coronary artery is blocked. It uses healthy blood vessels to create detours around narrowed or blocked arteries. Bypass surgery is usually an open-chest procedure.

- Cardiac catheterization. This is a common nonsurgical procedure which is used to help diagnose or locate artery, valve or heart muscle problems. During the procedure, a catheter is inserted and gently guided toward your heart while your doctor is watching the advancement of the catheter on a video monitor. The catheter position is changed multiple times throughout the test. Dye will be injected into the catheter in certain areas of your heart chamber and arteries to help visualize the areas. The intravascular ultrasound catheter will then be inserted to obtain higher resolution of the images for the assessment of coronary arteries, valves and post interventions such as angioplasty.

Task 5 **Theme-related discussion.**

Patients with severe coronary artery disease could develop heart failure, which urgently needs a heart transplant. The availability of donor organs is a fundamental prerequisite for running a transplantation program. Therefore, organ donation is a generous and worthwhile decision that can be a life-saving gift to multiple people.

Please watch the MOOC, think about it, and discuss the following questions with your partner.

1. What are the benefits of organ donation for medical science and practices?

2. What are the ethical and socio-cultural barriers to organ donation?

Part Ⅳ　Word Formation

kidney［英］肾

　ren-［拉］肾　renal *adj*. 肾的

　　renal duct（＝ureter）输尿管

　　renal function test（＝ kidney function test）肾功能试验

　　renal calculus /ˈkælkjʊləs/ 肾结石

　nephr(o)-［希］肾　nephric *adj*. 肾的（同 renal）

　　nephric duct 肾管

　　nephritis /nɪˈfraɪtɪs/ *n*. 肾炎（nephritic *adj*. 肾炎的）

　　nephric calculus /ˈkælkjələs/ 肾结石（同 renal calculus）

heart［英］心

　cardi(o)-［希］心　cardiac- *adj*. 心的

　　cardiac muscle 心肌

　　cardiac output 心排血量

　　cardioacceleratory /ˌkɑːdɪəʊækˈselərətəri/ *adj*. 心动加速的

lung［英］肺

　pulmo-，pulmon(o)-［拉］肺

　　pulmonary /ˈpʌlmənəri/ *adj*. 肺的

　　pulmogram /pʌlməˈgræm/ *n*. 肺部造影片

　　pulmonology /pʌlməˈnɒlədʒi/ *n*. 肺脏病学

lung［英］肺

　pneum(o)-［希］呼吸;肺;气;肺炎

　　pneumocardial /ˌnjuːməʊˈkɑːdɪəl/ *adj*. 肺心的,心肺的

　　pneumocephalus /ˌnjuːməʊˈsefələs/ *n*. 颅腔积气

　　pneumococcosis /ˌnjuːməʊkɒkəʊsɪs/ *n*. 肺炎球菌

cut［英］切(断)

　-tomy［希］切开术

　　oophorotomy /ˌɒfəˈrɒtəmi/ *n*. 卵巢切开术

ototomy /əˈtɒtəmi/ n. 耳切开术

urethrotomy /ˌjʊərɪˈθrɒtəmi/ n. 尿道切开术

swift [英] 快速

　tachy- [希] 速,快速

　　tachycardia /ˌtækɪˈkɑːdiə/ n. 心悸,心动过速

　　tachyphylaxis /ˌtækɪfəˈlæksɪs/ n. 快速免疫,快速脱敏,快速耐受

　　tachypnea /ˌtækɪpˈniə/ n. 呼吸急促

slow [英] 慢

　brady- [希] 缓,慢,迟钝

　　bradyarrhythmia /ˌbrædiəˈrɪθmiə/ n. 过缓性心律失常

　　bradyarthria /ˌbrædiˈɑːθriə/ n. 言语过缓

　　bradycardia /ˌbrædiˈkɑːdiə/ n. 心动过缓

Task 6 **Match each of the following terms with its definition.**

1　renin　　　　　A　abnormally slow breathing

2　nephron　　　 B　of or relating to the heart and the blood vessels

3　bradypnea　　 C　improper presence of air between the lungs and the chest wall

4　pneumothorax　D　an enzyme released by the kidneys

5　cardiovascular　E　a bacterium that invades the respiratory tract and is a major cause of pneumonia

6　pneumococcus　F　any of the minute urine-secreting tubules that form the functional unit of the kidneys

Task 7 **Fill in the blanks with words or phrases given in the box. Change the form where necessary.**

electrocardiogram	cardiac output	pulmonary ventilation	pneumonia
nephrology	nephritis	pneumoconiosis	tachycardia
renal pelvis	cardiotomy		

1. _____ is a measurement of the amount of blood pumped by each ventricle in one minute.

2. When you have _____, your heart beats faster than normal for a few seconds to a few hours.

3. Renal physiology is the study of kidney function, while _____ is the medical specialty concerned with kidney diseases.

4. An _____ represents a recording of the heart's electrical activity. It's a

common and painless test used to detect heart problems and monitor the heart's health quickly.

5. The inflammation of the _____ can be acute or chronic. Usually only one kidney is affected by the inflammation.

6. The most common respiratory diseases are chronic obstructive pulmonary disease, lung cancer, tuberculosis, and _____.

7. _____ is the act of breathing, which can be described as the movement of air into and out of the lungs. It comprises two major steps: inspiration and expiration.

8. The most frequently encountered types of _____, known as an occupational disease, are silicosis and coal miner's lung.

9. Acute interstitial _____, a common cause of acute kidney injury, is most often due to a hypersensitivity reaction to medications.

10. The suffix "otomy" means incision and "cardi" means heart, so the word _____ means a surgical incision into the heart.

Part V Fast Reading

How Does the Food Act in Your Digestive System

What happens to the food we eat? How does it get to the cells?

First the food goes into the digestive tract. It enters your body by the mouth, and travels down the gullet, a tube between your mouth and your stomach, then gets into your stomach, a big pouch at the top of your abdomen, and then into your small intestine and your large intestine.

But your food does not go along unchanged. Things keep happening to it every step of the way. When it comes into your body, the food is made up of millions and millions of big molecules held together in chunks. When the chunks are broken up physically by the teeth and the contraction of the stomach and intestines, the big molecules are broken up chemically by the digestive juices. From big protein molecules come somewhat smaller molecules of amino acids; from fats come fatty acids and glycerine; and from carbohydrates like the starches come the simple sugars. This whole process of physical and chemical break-down is called digestion.

The digested food molecules pass into the cells lining the inside of the intestine. These cells move them along into the tiny blood vessels which run all through the walls of the intestine. The blood then carries them to the cells in all parts of the body, and there, of course, they take part in the cells' metabolism. These molecules are broken down into very small ones. And with the energy released, you can run or read or go to the movies or do whatever you want to do.

But what causes the changes in the food as it goes through the digestive tract? And how is the blood able to carry it around?

On June 6, 1822, Alexis St. Martin, an eighteen years old French Canadian, stopped at a trading post on an island in Mackinac Straits, Michigan. Not more than a yard away from him, a gun went off by accident. Alexis was hit, and a big ragged hole was torn in his left side just below his chest.

In less than half an hour, Dr. William Beaumont, an Army surgeon stationed at Fort Mackinac, arrived to look after the wounded boy. The food Alexis has eaten for breakfast was pouring out of his stomach through the hole. Dr. Beaumont carefully removed all the shot and torn bits of clothing he could find in and around the wound. For seventeen days Alexis could not eat without losing the food through the hole in his stomach, so he had to be fed artificially. It was five weeks after the accident before he could digest normally. Dr. Beaumont tried to get the hole in Alexis' stomach to heal, but it would not. Finally he gave up and told Alexis he would have to have an operation. Alexis refused, so the hole stayed open.

Ten months passed before Alexis could walk around and do light work. A year after the accident, his wound had healed completely except for the two-and-a-half-inch hole into his stomach. By the winter of the next year, fold of the stomach wall had grown over the hole. It kept the food from coming out, but it still did not heal shut, though Alexis could now lead a normal life.

Dr. Beaumont realized that the hole in Alexis's stomach gave him a chance to find out by first hand observation a lot of things about digestion. The most important thing of all that Dr. Beaumont found out from Alexis's stomach was this: The food itself in the stomach made the muscles contract and the juices pour out; the food itself started up the changes which resulted in its own digestion.

But how did this work? That was still a mystery. Many years later a big step in finding the solution was taken by a famous scientist thousands of miles away in Russia. Ivan P. Pavlov set out to find out how the food made the stomach juice flow. He anesthetized a dog and made an opening in the outside wall of the dog's abdomen. Then he took a part of the dog's stomach and made a pouch out of it. This pouch had all the nerves and blood vessels that the rest of the stomach had. The food going in and out of the stomach could not get into the pouch. Pavlov made a separate opening in the pouch that led out through the hole in the abdominal wall.

Then Pavlov fed the dog. As soon as food got into its mouth, juice began to pour into the stomach. Some juice also poured into the pouch, and the scientist collected it in a little bottle through the opening in the abdominal wall. This experiment was one more proof that food itself starts its own digestion going. Pavlov showed that the presence of food in the mouth started nerve impulses that went to the brain and then to the cells of the stomach, which then secreted or poured out juices. When he cut the vagus nerves which bring impulses from the brain to the stomach, the dog's mouth could be stuffed with food yet no juices would be secreted in the stomach.

Just as you don't have to think in order to breathe, you don't have to think to digest. You can drink a glass of hot milk before you go to bed, and it will be digested long before morning. It is digested while you are asleep. We call such an activity of the body, which involves nerves and happens automatically, reflex. When food enters the mouth, a nerve impulse goes to the medulla. This is then "reflected" back by the nerves to the stomach. When the impulse reaches the stomach, the muscles contract and the cells secrete their juices. Physically and chemically, digestion has started. Pavlov also showed that the sight, the smell—even the thought—of food could start the reflexes going and the stomach secreting. At the thought of a nice thick steak, you could really say, "My stomach waters."

But these stomach juices are not poured out all at once. After the food reaches the stomach, more juices are secreted, particularly if the food contains lots of protein. Did you ever think why it is good to start a meal with soup? The proteins in the soup make your stomach secrete a lot of juice—all ready for the rest of the meal.

The protein-rich food gets partly digested by the first juices. Then this partly digested food stimulates certain stomach cells to secrete—not more juices into the stomach, but a substance called gastrin into the blood. It is as if somebody knocked on the front door as a signal for someone else to run out of the back door. Now gastrin is a hormone, and hormones are chemical substances that make things happen in specific parts of the body. In this case, gastrin makes the stomach's juice-secreting cells pour out more juices. It is as if the person who went out of the back door ran around the corner and signaled someone in another house to turn on the water faucets.

From the stomach, the food travels on down the digestive tract. It is out of the stomach in four or five hours. As it enters the intestine—it's in semi-liquid form now—it starts a whole new set of cells secreting. Some of these cells are in the intestine itself. Others are in two big glands, the liver and the pancreas; their juices reach the food in the intestine through little tubes. Some of these cells secrete because of nerve impulses, others because of hormones. It takes juices five different places—the mouth, the stomach, the intestines, the liver and the pancreas—to get your food broken down into molecules small enough to be moved by the cells of the intestine into the blood vessels.

Task 8 **Read the passage and decide whether the statements are true or false. If it is true, write "T". If it is not, write "F".**

1. The digestive tract is composed of the mouth, the gullet, the stomach, the small intestine and the large intestine.   (   )

2. The whole process of digestion produces amino acids from protein, fatty acids and glycerine from fats and the simple sugars from the carbohydrates.   (   )

3. The digested food molecules pass into the cells lining the inside of the intestine.

But they are not involved in the cells' metabolism.　　　　　　　　（　　）

4. What Dr. Beaumont found out from Alexis's stomach was that the food in the stomach made the muscles contract and the juices pour out，causing the food itself to start up the changes which result in its own digestion.　　　　　　　　（　　）

5. Ivan P. Pavlov's studies aimed to find out where the stomach juice came from.

　　　　　　　　（　　）

Task 9 **Please read the passage again and write a two-hundred-word synopsis.**

Part Ⅵ　Translation

Task 10 **Please analyze the following sentences and then put them into Chinese.**

1. The nutritive blood flow to all but the alveolar structures comes from the bronchial circulation，which originates from the aorta and upper intercostal arteries and receives about 1 per cent of the cardiac output.

2. The arteries down to the level of the subsegmental airways（2 mm diameter）are thin-walled，predominantly elastic vessels.

3. These vessels subdivide further as they enter the renal parenchyma and create interlobar arteries that course toward the renal cortex.

医学翻译技巧

标题写作与翻译技巧

标题是文章的重要组成部分，是整篇论文内容的高度概括，标题突出论文中心，便于检索。因受限于字数的要求，标题的书写应用词准确、简明扼要、层次清晰。从语法结构来说，文摘标题常采用短语形式，亦可用句子形式。

短语形式的文摘标题多用名词短语，常见如下：

例1　Aortic Valve Insufficiency in a 45-year-old Male

一名45岁男性二尖瓣关闭不全病例讨论

结构：单名词+介词短语。名词表明研究主题，介词短语引出更为详细的信息。

例2　Benefits and limitations of serological assays in HIV infection
在 HIV 感染中进行血清学检测的益处和局限性的<u>研究</u>

结构：名词 and 名词+介词短语

例3　Surgery versus Conservative Care for Persistent Sciatica Lasting 4 to 12 Months
对持续4至12个月坐骨神经痛病人进行手术与保守治疗的对比<u>研究</u>

结构：名词 versus 名词+介词短语

注意，例2和例3属于双名词+介词短语结构，前者用来表示两者之间的联系，后者用来表示两个事物之间的对比关系。

例4　Analysis of Surface Proteins of Mouse Lung Carcinoma Using Monoclonal Antibodies
单克隆抗体对小鼠肺癌表面蛋白的<u>分析研究</u>

结构：名词+非谓语动词短语
如果名词短语形式的标题过长，可加副标题，如：

例5　The relationship between rumination and NSSI：A systematic review and meta-analysis
反刍思维与非自杀性自伤的关系：系统综述和元分析

试比较：A systematic review and meta-analysis of the relationship between rumination and NSSI

采用副标题形式既可避免多层冗长的偏正结构短语，又有突出论文中心内容、研究方法或者病例数的作用，再如：

例6　Echocardiography in transcatheter closure of ventricule septal deficit：A practical study of 62 cases
62例心脏超声指导室间隔缺损介入治疗的应用<u>研究</u>

在写作与翻译标题时，还需要注意对病例数的处理。在国外医学期刊中，即使病例数很大，有时也不被列入标题，只是在摘要正文一开始就说明病例数（见例7）。所以在汉译英时，病例数字有时可删去不译（见例8）。

例7　Heparin Therapy：A randomized prospective study
Eighty patients were assigned randomly either to continuous or to intermittent heparin therapy ...
肝素疗法的前瞻性随机研究
80例肝素治疗患者随机分配到连续性或间断性给药（两个组）……

例8　慢性胃炎分类的探讨（附71例分析）

Evaluation of Classification of Chronic Gastritis

除短语外,标题还可用句子来表述,这在国外医学期刊中也很常见。

例 9　Early surgery improves cure of aneurysms-induced oculomotor palsy
　　　　早期手术可以改善动脉瘤引起的动眼肌麻痹

试比较:Effect of early surgery on cure of aneurysms-induced oculomotor palsy

采用句子形式的文摘标题可突出医学论文的中心信息,而短语形式的标题并未明确说明早期手术的作用,而此"作用"恰恰是论文的重点内容。

另外,国外医学期刊英文标题一般直截了当,诸如 "thought of ...""observation on ..." "study of ..." 和 "investigation of ..." 等短语很少出现。因此在汉译英标题时,"关于""研究""报告""观察"等字样常可省略不译,参看前面的例1、例2、例4、例6。

再如:

例 10　(Study of) Toxic effects of benzene on leucocytes
　　　　苯对白细胞毒性作用的研究

该标题中括号里的 study 无实质意义,可以省略。

论文的标题还要注意省略谦虚客套用语。中文标题中的"刍议""初步研究"等谦虚字眼,译成英文时往往省略不译。

例 11　Acupuncture anesthesia for open-heart operation
　　　　心脏手术针刺麻醉初步报告

试比较:A preliminary report on acupuncture anesthesia for open-heart operation

preliminary 属谦虚客套用语,在科技论文中可省略。

最后,期刊论文标题在大小写方面也有各自不同的要求,总结如下:

(1)每一个字母都大写。

例 12　WEIGHT LOSS IN ALZHEIMER'S DISEASE
　　　　阿尔茨海默病患者体重减轻

(2)除第一个单词的首字母大写外,其余均小写。

例 13　Inflammatory bowel disease in the older patient
　　　　老年患者中的感染性肠道疾病

(3)除虚词(冠词、连接词、介词等)外,每个词的首字母都大写。

例 14　White-Coat Hypertension：the Neglected Subgroup in Hypertension
　　　　白大衣高血压：高血压的被忽视亚组

(4)标题中间有破折号时,其后面的冠词、介词通常也要大写。

例 15　New Insights into Erectile Dysfunction—A Practical Approach
　　　　勃起功能障碍的新观点：一种实用方法研究

(5)标题中间有冒号时,其后面的冠词、介词通常也要大写。

例 16　Hepcidin and Anemia：A Tight Relationship
　　　　铁调素与贫血的密切关系

Task 11 **Rewrite the following titles.**

1. Investigation of increase of endurance of muscular strength of middle school students

_____

2. 58 Artificial Joint Replacements Were Performed in Patients Who Had Type Ⅱ Diabetes

_____

3. A Systematic Review of Psychosocial Factors Affecting Parental Report of Symptoms in Children

_____

4. Heart Disease after Diabetes：a Follow-up Study

_____

5. A preliminary study of antibody-dependent enhancement of coronavirus

_____

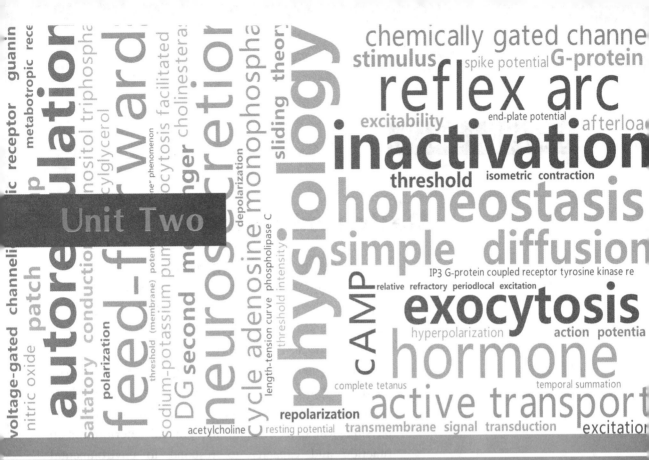

Physiology

✓课文音频
✓听力音频
✓在线课程
✓课件申请

Cells and Aging

homeostatic /ˌhəʊmɪəʊˈstætɪk/ *adj.*
稳态的

geriatrics /ˌdʒerɪˈætrɪks/ *n.* （作单数
用）老年病学

metabolism /məˈtæbəlɪzəm/ *n.* 新陈
代谢
homeostasis /ˌhəʊmɪəʊˈsteɪsɪs/ *n.* 稳
态，内稳态

extracellular /ˌekstrəˈseljʊlə/ *adj.*
（位于或发生于）细胞外的
collagen /ˈkɒlədʒən/ *n.* 胶原质
tendon /ˈtendn/ *n.* ［解］腱

atherosclerosis /ˌæθərəʊsklɪəˈrəʊsɪs/
n. 动脉粥样硬化
elastin /ɪˈlæstɪn/ *n.* 弹性蛋白

glucose /ˈgluːkəʊs/ *n.* 葡萄糖

Aging is a normal process accompanied by a progressive alteration of the body's homeostatic adaptive responses; the specialized branch of medicine that deals with the medical problems and care of elderly persons is called geriatrics.

The obvious characteristics of aging are well known: graying and loss of hair, loss of teeth, wrinkling of skin, decreased muscle mass, and increased fat deposits. The physiological signs of aging are gradual deterioration in function and capacity to respond to environmental stresses. Metabolism slows, as does the ability to maintain a constant internal environment（homeostasis）in response to changes in temperature, diet, and oxygen supply. These signs of aging are related to a net decrease in the number of cells in the body and to the dysfunctioning of the cells that remain.

The extracellular components of tissues also change with age. Collagen fibers, responsible for the strength in tendons, increase in number and change in quality with aging. These changes in the collagen of arterial walls are as much responsible for their loss of extensibility as are the deposits associated with atherosclerosis, the deposition of fatty materials in arterial walls. Elastin, another extracellular component, is responsible for the elasticity of blood vessels and skin. It thickens, fragments, and acquires a greater affinity for calcium with age-changes that may also be associated with the development of atherosclerosis.

Glucose, the most abundant sugar in the body, may play a role in the aging process. According to one hypothesis, glucose is added, haphazardly, to proteins inside and outside cells, forming irreversible cross-links between adjacent protein molecules. As a person ages, more cross-links are formed, and this probably contributes to the stiffening and loss of elasticity that occurs in aging tissues.

Although many millions of new cells normally are produced each minute, several kinds of cells in the body — heart cells, skeletal muscle fibers, nerve cells — cannot be replaced. Experiments have shown that many other cell types have only a limited capability to divide. Cells grown outside the body divide only a certain number of times and then stop. The number of divisions correlates with the donor's age and with the normal life span of the different species from which the cells are obtained. These observations provide strong evidence for the hypothesis that cessation of **mitosis** is a normal, genetically programmed event. According to this view, an "aging" gene is part of the genetic blueprint at birth, and it turns on at a preprogrammed time, slowing down or halting processes vital to life.

mitosis /mɪˈtəʊsɪs/ n. (细胞的)有丝分裂

Another theory of aging is the free **radical** theory. Free radicals are electrically charged molecules that have an unpaired electron. Such molecules are unstable and highly reactive and can easily damage proteins. Some effects are wrinkled skin, stiff joints, and hardened arteries. Free radicals may also damage DNA. Among the factors that produce free radicals are air pollution, radiation, and certain foods we eat. Other substances in the diet such as vitamin E, vitamin C, beta-carotene, and **selenium** are **antioxidants** and inhibit free radical formation. The free radical theory of aging is **bolstered** by two recent discoveries. Strains of fruit flies bred for longevity produce larger-than-normal amounts of an **enzyme** called **superoxide dismutase**, which functions to neutralize free radicals. Also, injection of genes that lead to production of superoxide dismutase into fruit fly **embryos** prolongs their average lifetime.

radical /ˈrædɪkəl/ n. [化]基
free radical 自由基,游离基

selenium /səˈliːniəm/ n. 硒
antioxidant /ˌæntiˈɒksɪdənt/ n. 抗氧化剂
bolster /ˈbəʊlstə/ v. 支持

enzyme /ˈenzaɪm/ n. 酶
superoxide /ˌsjuːpəˈɒksaɪd/ n. 过氧化物
dismutase /dɪsˈmjuːteɪs/ n. 歧化酶
embryo /ˈembriəʊ/ n. 胚胎

Whereas some theories of aging explain the process at the cellular level, others concentrate on regulatory mechanisms operating within the entire organism. For example, the immune system, which manufactures antibodies against foreign invaders, may start to attack the body's own cells. This autoimmune response might be caused by changes in the surfaces of cells, causing antibodies to attach and mark the cell for destruction. As surface changes in cells increase, the autoimmune response intensifies, producing the well-known signs of aging.

Task 1 **Find out the answers to the following questions and then compare your answers with a partner.**

    1. How is aging defined?

    2. What are the physiological signs of aging?

    3. According to the text, what contributes to the elasticity of blood vessels and skin?

    4. Is it true that all kinds of cells can be replaced?

    5. What are the theories of aging proposed in this text?

Part II Listening

Task 2 **You will hear 20 words or phrases which will be read three times. Write them down on the blanks and check with your partner after you finish.**

1. _____ 2. _____ 3. _____ 4. _____

5. _____ 6. _____ 7. _____ 8. _____

9. _____ 10. _____ 11. _____ 12. _____

13. _____ 14. _____ 15. _____ 16. _____

17. _____ 18. _____ 19. _____ 20. _____

You are going to hear a passage which will be read three times. Take some notes while you are listening to the passage and then answer the following questions.

1. What does physiology aim to do?

_____

2. What is the significance of research in physiology?

_____

3. What can be regarded as fundamental processes of the body?

_____

Part Ⅲ　Oral Presentation and Discussion

Task 4 Read the following passage and make an oral presentation.

Psychological Aspects of Aging

Aging does not increase the risk of developing a mental illness such as depression or anxiety. Some disorders, such as bipolar disorder or schizophrenia, typically begin in early adulthood and persist into later life. Other disorders such as major depression or phobias can begin at any point in the lifespan. The American Association of Geriatric Psychiatry estimates that about 20% of the population over age 55 experience some type of mental disorder, although the prevalence of the most severe forms of these disorders, such as schizophrenia or bipolar disorder, is much smaller. However, evidence clearly shows that mental illness is not part of normal aging. Older adults with untreated mental illness have worse health status and physical functioning, reduced social connections, and more stressed caregivers. For these reasons, mental illnesses in older adults present an important public health issue.

Underdiagnosis and undertreatment are systemic problems for older adults. A number of reasons appear to contribute to the under-detection and treatment of mental health problems in older adults, including stigma and related reluctance to seek help, an assumption that symptoms are part of normal aging, and presentation of purely physical symptoms. Most older adults respond well to treatment when the illness or disorder is detected early.

Approximately 25% of older adults with mental health or substance abuse disorders receive mental health treatment. Older adults tend to receive mental health treatment in the primary care setting rather than with mental health specialists. Although older adults report less experience using mental health services than do younger people, one study found that they are more open to referrals for mental health care from multiple sources and have more positive attitudes about mental health services than do younger adults.

In addition to biological and genetic elements that can cause mental illness, a number of other etiological factors may also relate to the onset of a mental illness. Such factors include alcohol, prescription and over-the-counter medications and herbal remedies, and nutritional deficiencies. Physical illnesses or injuries and lack of exercise can also increase the risk of experiencing a mental illness. Older adults experience losses of loved ones or of meaningful activities, as well as illnesses, more frequently than their younger peers; such stressful events increase the risk of developing certain types of mental health disorders.

Absent of disease-related pathology, the overall size of the brain decreases with age, accompanied by a loss of neurons. These changes develop gradually over the lifespan; in fact, the time of greatest neuronal loss occurs between 2 months of age to 18 years. Even late in life, the cerebral cortex remains somewhat adaptable, allowing for ongoing cognitive and emotional development. In general, older adults experience slowing of cerebral processing and deficits in recall compared to younger adults. However, accumulated knowledge and experience may serve to counterbalance these declines.

Age-related declines in memory function exist in multiple types of memory, including recollection, declarative memory, episodic memory, and working memory. Other memory forms are less affected by age such as familiarity, semantic knowledge, and nondeclarative memory. Declarative memory refers to memories of events or facts that can be consciously recalled; nondeclarative memory refers to acquired skills or other unconscious memory. Underlying causes of age-related memory deficits include overall slowing in ability to process information, leading to difficulty in retrieving memories quickly, as well as concomitant changes in sensory perception, which can impair information processing. Various types of intervention show some success in improving memory, including cardiovascular and cognitive exercise and various memory training strategies.

Abnormal memory impairment exists when it disrupts normal daily functioning, most commonly attributable to dementia. Dementia affects 6%~8% of men and women over 65 and 50% of people 85 or older. Few types of dementia are reversible, although certain types of treatment slow disease progression and manage some of the symptoms. The most prevalent dementia symptoms include gradual decrease in memory, attention, and judgment; disorientation; communication and word finding difficulty; inappropriate social behavior; and personality changes. Alzheimer's disease, followed by vascular dementia, are the most prevalent forms; dementia often accompanies other conditions such as Parkinson's disease, Huntington's disease, alcoholism, and AIDS.

Task 5 Theme-related discussion.

As we all know, the Nobel Prize in Physiology or Medicine awards the person who has made the most important discovery within a specific domain. Tu Youyou received the Nobel Prize at the age of 85, an age when scientists possess much more knowledge, experience and achievements.

Please watch the MOOC, think about it, and discuss the following questions with your partner.

1. Why did Tu Youyou attract so much attention when she was awarded the Nobel Prize in Physiology or Medicine?

2. How did Tu Youyou's discovery of artemisinin embody "Never too old to learn"?

Part Ⅳ　Word Formation

against［英］对抗

　anti-［希］相反；反对；抵抗

　　antioxidant /ˌæntɪˈɒksɪdənt/ n. 抗氧化剂

　　antibody /ˈæntɪˌbɒdi/ n. 抗体

　　antiallergic /ˌæntiəˈlɜːdʒɪk/ n. 抗变应性的

same［英］同,等

　homeo-，homo-［希］相同的

　　homeostasis /ˌhəʊmiəˈsteɪsɪs/ n. 稳态,内稳态

　　homeotherapy /ˌhəʊmiəˈθerəpi/ n. 顺势疗法

　　homogeneity /ˌhɒməˈdʒɑːniːəti/ n. 同种,同质

origin［英］原

　-gen［希］原

　　antigen /ˈæntɪdʒən/ n. 抗原

　　glycogen /ˈɡlaɪkədʒen/ n. 糖原

　　pathogen /ˈpæθədʒ(ə)n/ n. 病原体

　　collagen /ˈkɒlədʒen/ n. 胶原质

stiff　［英］硬

　-sclerosis［希］硬化

　　arteriosclerosis /ɑːˌtɪəriəʊskləˈrəʊsɪs/ n. 动脉硬化

　　cardiosclerosis /ˌkɑːdiəʊskləˈrəʊsɪs/ n. 心肌硬化

　　osteosclerosis /ˌɒstiəʊskləˈrəʊsɪs/ n. 骨硬化,骨质过密

　　atherosclerosis /ˌæθərəʊskləˈrəʊsɪs/ n. 动脉粥样硬化

　-ostomy［希］造口术,造瘘术,吻合术

　　cholecystoduodenostomy /ˌkɒlɪsɪstəˌdjʊ(ː)ədɪˈnɒstəmi/ n. 胆囊十二指肠吻合术

　　gastrostomy /ɡæsˈtrɒstəmi/ n. 胃造口术

　　neocystostomy /ˌniəʊsɪsˈtɒstəmi/ n. 膀胱再造口术

mind［英］智力,精神,心理

　psych(o)-［希］精神,心理

　　psychedelic /ˌsaɪkəˈdelɪk/ adj. 致幻的　　n. 致幻剂

　　psychiatry /saɪˈkaɪətri/ n. 精神病学

　　psychotherapy /ˌsaɪkəʊˈθerəpi/ n. 心理治疗

water［英］水

　hydr(o)-［希］水，积液,氢

hydrogymnastic /ˌhaɪdrəudʒɪmˈnæstɪk/ *adj.* 水中运动的

hydroappendix /ˌhaɪdrəuəˈpendɪks/ *n.* 阑尾积水

hydrocholesterol /ˌhaɪdrəukəˈlestərəul/ *n.* 氢化胆固醇

Task 6 **Match each of the following terms with its definition.**

1	collagen	A	accumulation of urine in the kidney
2	hydronephrosis	B	abnormal thickening and loss of elasticity in the arterial walls
3	antibacterial	C	of uniform quality, structure, or composition
4	arteriosclerosis	D	agents that prevent or treat bipolar disorder, a mental illness
5	antimanic drugs	E	any of a class of extracellular proteins that is abundant in bone, tendons, cartilage, and connective tissue
6	homogeneous	F	effective against bacteria

Task 7 **Fill in the blanks with words or phrases given in the box. Change the form where necessary.**

homeostasis	hydrogen	antibiotic	hydrophobia
antifebrile	glycogen	homotransplantation	psychiatrist
psychoanalysis	gastrostomy		

1. If the victim of a dog-bite is not treated in time, _____ , or fear of water may occur, which will result in the inability to swallow water.

2. _____ refers to moving tissues or organs from one individual to another of the same species.

3. Medicines that fight bacterial infections are called _____ . They work to clear up infections either by killing bacteria or stopping their growth.

4. Psychologists and _____ are two key types of mental health experts. But their training differs, as do the tools for treatment they have at their disposal, and often their theoretical orientation as well.

5. The doctor prescribed an _____ medication to help reduce the patient's fever.

6. A _____ feeding tube insertion is the placement of a feeding tube through the skin and the stomach wall.

7. Body temperature _____ keeps the body's temperature stable at around 98.6 degrees F and helps offset the risks of heat exhaustion or hypothermia.

8. _____ is the body's stored form of glucose, which is sugar. It is made from

several connected glucose molecules and is your body's primary and preferred source of energy.

9. In biology, _____ plays a crucial role in various biochemical and physiological processes. It is the third most abundant element (9.5% by mass) in the human body, after oxygen (65%) and carbon (18.5%).

10. _____, first popularized by the famous psychologist Sigmund Freud, is based on the belief that all humans have deep, unconscious beliefs, thoughts, memories, and desires.

Part V   Fast Reading

10 Easy Steps to a Healthier Heart

Keep your heart healthy and reduce your heart attack risk with these simple tips.

Even if you follow just the first seven tips below (and don't smoke, of course), you'll reduce the chance of having a heart attack by as much as 90 percent compared to a typical person of your age!

1. Walk 30 minutes a day every day, and then call someone. Walking a half-hour a day decreases the risk of having a heart attack by about 30 percent. I've found if you succeed at walking daily, you can also succeed at doing other things to improve health. If you skip, you'll start compromising health in other ways too. Calling someone every day is crucial; that's the real commitment. Find a person who's supportive and will not nag but will call if you haven't called her. And by the way, it usually is a "her." Men tend to be lousy at this!

2. Know your blood pressure and do whatever it takes to get it down to 115/75. Your blood pressure number may be even more important than your cholesterol. And you can lower it yourself. The best way? Getting a little exercise and losing some belly fat. Why belly fat? The omentum is what hangs over the stomach. The

fat that's stored there feeds the kidney, liver and other vital organs. Here's the hypothesis: When you gain weight, you add fat inside the relatively rigid "kidney capsule." This fat pushes on the kidney, so it says, "Hey, I need more blood pressure to drive blood through because I'm getting squeezed by the fat." So it releases hormones that cause increased blood pressure. When you lose a little of that fat, even with just a few pounds of weight loss, your blood pressure goes down really fast. Cutting back on salt may help, but for some people reducing sugar and saturated fat in the diet may help even more. Recently I coached a patient (he'll be on the PBS special You on a Diet coming in March) whose blood pressure started at 160/100, but he didn't have any arterial disease. In seven weeks, he had his blood pressure down to 115/75 with just weight loss, walking and decreasing sugar and saturated fat in his diet. But if your blood pressure is over 140/90 and you're not going to do these things reliably, then you should probably go on blood-pressure medication. New drugs can reduce blood pressure without major side effects.

3. Eat an ounce of nuts a day. Nuts raise HDL good cholesterol and decrease inflammation. But they have a heart benefit independent of those too. We're not sure why. Nuts have healthy omega-3 fatty acids, healthy protein and some fiber. And this tip is easy to do! Nuts that are raw, fresh and unsalted have the most benefit. You can develop a taste for them if you give them a chance. But if you want to roast, say, (shelled) walnuts, put them in the oven at 350 degrees for about 9 minutes. If you do it yourself, it won't cause any bad fats or dangerous chemical acrylamides to form.

4. Learn your HDL number and do what you can to raise it to 50. For women, some believe a high HDL is more important than a lower LDL. We have no idea why, but study after study shows that the higher the number, the better (50 is fine). Easy ways you can increase it: exercise; have one drink a day; eat healthy fats, such as olive and canola oil and nuts. Talk to your doctor about niacin, which raises HDL but can have side effects. Ask, too, about pantothenic acid, or vitamin B_5, which may also help. While the main function of statin drugs is to lower LDL, some also raise HDL.

5. Eat 10 tablespoons of tomato sauce a week. This is one of

my favorite tips. Tomato sauce is loaded with blood-pressure-slashing potassium. We're not talking about salty, fatty sauces, or serving with a huge portion of pasta. Keep it simple and healthy, and get a great benefit.

6. Floss your teeth regularly. Avoiding periodontal disease prevents inflammation in the arteries, which helps you head off heart disease. Most people don't know that your oral health affects all your arterial health, and that includes blood flow to the heart and sexual organs, and maybe even wrinkles on your skin.

7. Eat no more than 20 grams of saturated fat a day and as little trans fat as possible. Saturated fat and trans fats lead to inflammation in the arteries. A cinnamon roll may have 7 grams of saturated fat. A 4-ounce slice of roast pork tenderloin has about 4 grams. Trans fats (partially hydrogenated oils), found in many processed and baked foods, are probably at least as bad as saturated fats, and maybe a little worse.

8. Read labels and throw out all food that has sugar in the first five ingredients. Don't be fooled by foods that are low in fat but high in sugar. The sugar causes inflammation. And if you eat more sugar than you need, it gets morphed into omentum fat, that dangerous fat around the belly. For a while in the 1990s, many people used "low fat" salad dressings that turned out to be loaded with calorie-laden sugar. And those dressings didn't contain any good fats like olive oil, which are beneficial. Healthy fats are better than empty sugar calories. (Because the sugar in fruit is in a complex carbohydrate, it's usually fine.)

9. Have a glass of wine or beer today. We're not sure why; there may be an anti-inflammatory effect. But it's a consistent finding that teetotalers have a higher risk of heart disease than people who drink a little, and people who drink a lot have little heart disease but tend to die of cancer. Seven drinks on Friday night is not the same as one every night! We know there are serious dangers to drinking, but still, any kind of alcohol in moderation is good for arteries.

10. Eat 9 servings of colorful fruits and vegetables a day. That comes with a lot of fiber. You'll adjust in 2 to 6 weeks. Make sure you wash fresh produce carefully and thoroughly. There are farmers' markets all over the country now. If you try fresh locally grown veggies prepared well, you'll be amazed at how good they taste.

Task 8 Read the passage and decide whether the statements are true or false. If it is true, write "T". If it is not, write "F".

1. If you skip the daily 30-minute walk, you'll start compromising health in other ways too.   (   )

2. Getting a little exercise and cutting back on salt is the best way to lower your blood pressure.   (   )

3. Your oral health affects all your arterial health.   (   )

4. Eat foods that are low in fat but high in sugar, and you will get little fat around your belly.   (   )

5. People who don't drink have a higher risk of heart disease than those who drink a little.   (   )

Task 9 Please read the passage again and write a two-hundred-word synopsis.

Part VI   Translation

Task 10 Please analyze the following sentences and then put them into Chinese.

1. These changes in the collagen of arterial walls are as much responsible for their loss of extensibility as are the deposits associated with atherosclerosis, the deposition of fatty materials in arterial walls.

_____

2. As a person ages, more cross-links are formed, and this probably contributes to the stiffening and loss of elasticity that occurs in aging tissues.

_____

3. These observations provide strong evidence for the hypothesis that cessation of mitosis is a normal, genetically programmed event.

_____

时 态

英文摘要类型各不相同,摘要中常用的时态也不相同。资料性摘要是当前医学英语论文摘要的主要形式。资料性摘要一般包括:(1) 研究目的、研究背景;(2) 研究过程和方法;(3) 研究结果;(4) 研究结论以及对未来的展望。其中最主要的内容是研究过程、方法和结果,相应的英语时态运用比较丰富,现分述如下:

介绍论文研究的背景、现状及尚待解决的问题,常用一般现在时或现在完成时。

例1 The toxic effects of acute or chronic use of alcohol on cerebral and hepatic function have long been recognized, but it has been thought that the heart is not similarly affected.

暴饮或长期饮酒对脑及肝脏的毒性作用已久为人知,但人们一直认为对心脏并无类似的影响。

说明研究的内容和目的、资料的来源和收集方法,研究的起止时间和主要结果,描述过去研究过程中进行的活动,常用一般过去时或过去完成时,而研究结论常用一般现在时。下面是一篇医学论文摘要的目的、方法、结果和结论部分。

例2 **Abstract**

Objective:Systemic sclerosis (SSc) is a connective tissue disease characterized by tissue fibrosis that reflects an imbalance between collagen production and degradation. Matrix metalloproteinases (MMPs) are a family of endopeptidases involved in the remodeling of extracellular matrix (ECM). This activity is controlled by tissue inhibitors of MMP (TIMPs). Aim of this study was the evaluation of MMP-9/TIMP-1 and MMP-2/TIMP-2 systems in patients with SSc.

Design and Method:Search Light Human MMP Array 1 was used to measure MMPs and TIMPs in 32 SSc patients and 32 matched healthy controls.

Results:SSc patients showed higher values of both MMP-9 and TIMP-1 in comparison with controls. The patients with anticentromere antibodies (ACA) positivity showed higher values of MMPs and TIMPs in comparison with either controls or the patients with anti-Sc170-positive antibodies.

Conclusion:Results of this investigation suggest that SSc patients with ACA positivity, after a primary fibrogenetic noxa, react with a more abundant release of MMP/TIMP, whereas patients with anti-Sc170 antibody show a normal response.

值得注意的是,摘要里提及的研究目的(aim of this study)是指作者于研究前所确定的研究目标,它与"本文目的"(aim of this paper)是两个不同的概念,语义意图也不同,所以研究目的用过去时表达,常用的句型有:

The purpose of this study (investigation) was to ...

The study was designed to ...

The objective of this study was to ...

The present study was undertaken to ...

The study reported here was undertaken ...

而本文目的用一般现在时表达：

The purpose of this paper is to ...

如果要表示研究过程开始前已经做过的工作或存在的状态,可用过去完成时。作者在做完了研究工作后得出的结论,无论是肯定的还是否定的,都用一般现在时表示,也有用一般过去时叙述结论的。此时这两种时态的语用意义不同,表达了作者两种截然不同的语义意图。用一般现在时表示作者认为该结论具有普遍意义,用一般过去时表示该结论不具有普遍意义,只是当时的研究结果而已。

例 3　结论：罗-阿氏窦变化是形成壁内结石的基本条件,胆囊切除是有效的方法。
We conclude that the presence of the Rokitansky Aschoff Sinus is the basis of the occurrence of the intramural gallstones and cholesystectomy is an effective treatment.

例 4　类叶升麻甘具有神经保护作用,能对抗 MPTP 诱导的 C57 小鼠的神经损伤,其机制可能与上调的 α-突触核蛋白水平有关。
Acteoside might be able to protect C57 mice against MPTP-induced neuronal damage. The neuroprotective effect might be associated with the up-regulation of α-synuclein level.

常用的表示结论的句型有：

The results show/suggest ...

We conclude that ... /It is concluded that ...

The results presented in the paper illustrate ...

This analysis suggests that ...

The results show ...

This case illustrates that ...

We recommend that ... be ... /It is recommended that ... be ...

描写对未来的展望,提及今后要做的工作及预期的结果和价值时,需用一般将来时。

例 5　As greater clinical correlation is obtained, the usefulness of thyroglobulin determination will increase.
随着人们对甲状腺蛋白水平与临床相关性有关知识的了解,测定甲状腺球蛋白的必要性也在提高。

Task 11 Complete the following sentences with the proper forms of the words given in the brackets.

1. Many physiological reactions _____ (aim) at preserving a constant physical and chemical internal environment (homeostasis).

2. The aim of this study _____ (be, evaluate) the future direction of green tea and the possibility of using green tea as a potential chemopreventive agent for stomach cancer intervention.

3. The purpose of this paper _____ (be, provide) an analysis of gender-based disparities in hypertension and cardiovascular disease care in ambulatory practices across the United States.

4. We therefore _____ (investigate) the associations of intake of dairy products, calcium, and vitamin D with the incidence of hypertension in a prospective cohort of 28 886 US women aged ≥45 years.

5. The model group _____ (show) remarkable depression of GLUT2 protein expression, _____ (compare) with the control group.

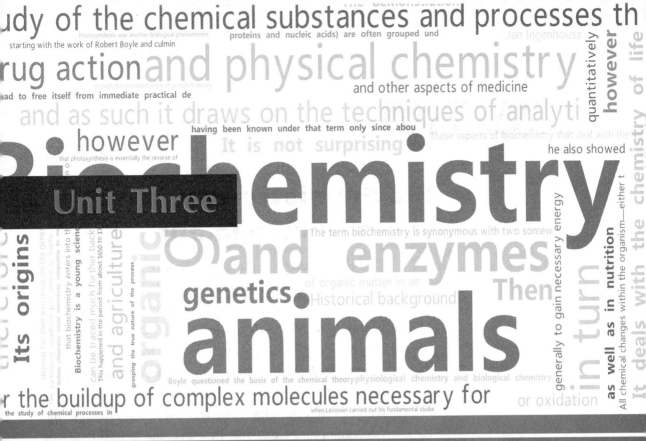

Biochemistry

✓课文音频
✓听力音频
✓在线课程
✓课件申请

Biochemistry and Human Development

Biochemistry is the application of chemistry to the study of biological processes at the cellular and molecular level. It emerged as a distinct discipline around the beginning of the 20th century when scientist combined chemistry, physiology and biology to investigate the chemistry of living systems. In a sense, biochemistry is both a life science and a chemical science. It uses the methods of chemistry, physics, molecular biology and immunology to study the structure and behavior of the complex molecules found in biological material and the ways those molecules interact to form cells, tissues and whole organism. It covers a broad range of cellular functions from gene transcription to the structure and function of macromolecules.

Biochemistry has become the foundation for understanding all biological processes. It has provided explanations for the causes of many diseases in humans, animals and plants. Our understanding of biochemistry has had and will continue to have extensive effects on many aspects of human endeavor. First, biochemistry is an intrinsically beautiful and fascinating body of knowledge. We now know the essence and many of the details of the most fundamental processes in biochemistry, such as how a single molecule of DNA replicates to generate two identical copies of itself and how the sequence of bases in a DNA molecule determines the sequence of amino acids in an encoded protein. Our ability to describe these processes in detailed, mechanistic terms places a firm chemical foundation under other biological sciences. Moreover, the realization that we can

transcription /træns'krɪpʃən/ n. [生物学] 转录，信使核糖核酸的形成
macromolecule /ˌmækrəʊ'mɒləkjuːl/ n. 大分子，高分子

intrinsically /ɪn'trɪnsɪkəli/ adv. 内在地；固有地，本征地，实质地

replicate /'replɪkeɪt/ v. 复制

amino /'æmɪnəʊ/ adj. 氨基的
encode /ɪn'kəʊd/ vt. 编码

understand essential life processes, such as the transmission of hereditary information, as chemical structures and their reactions has significant philosophical implications. What does it mean, biochemically, to be human? What are the biochemical differences between a human being, a chimpanzee, a mouse, and a fruit fly? Are we more similar than we are different?

Second, biochemistry is greatly influencing medicine and other fields. The molecular lesions causing **sickle-cell anemia**, **cystic fibrosis**, **hemophilia**, and many other genetic diseases have been **elucidated** at the biochemical level. Some of the molecular events that contribute to cancer development have been identified. An understanding of the underlying defects opens the door to the discovery of effective therapies. Biochemistry makes possible the rational design of new drugs, including specific **inhibitors** of enzymes required for the replication of viruses such as human **immunodeficiency** virus (HIV). Genetically engineered bacteria or other organisms can be used as "factories" to produce valuable proteins such as insulin and stimulators of blood-cell development.

Biochemistry is also contributing richly to clinical diagnostics. For example, elevated levels of **telltale** enzymes in the blood reveal whether a patient has recently had a **myocardial infarction** (heart attack). DNA probes are coming into play in the precise diagnosis of inherited disorders, infectious diseases, and cancers. Agriculture, too, is benefiting from advances in biochemistry with the development of more effective, environmentally safer **herbicides** and **pesticides** and the creation of genetically engineered plants that are, for example, more resistant to insects. All of these endeavors are being accelerated by the advances in genomic sequencing.

Third, advances in biochemistry are enabling researchers to tackle some of the most exciting questions in biology and medicine. How does a fertilized egg give rise to cells as different as those in muscle, brain, and liver? How do the senses work? What are the molecular

sickle-cell anemia 镰状细胞血症
cystic /'sɪstɪk/ adj. 胞囊的;膀胱的;胆囊的
fibrosis /faɪ'brəʊsɪs/ n. 纤维症
hemophilia /ˌhiːməʊ'fɪliə/ n. 血友病
elucidate /i'luːsɪdeɪt/ v. 阐明,说明

inhibitor /ɪn'hɪbɪtə/ n. 抑制剂
immunodeficiency /ˌɪmjuːnəʊdɪ'fɪʃənsi/ n. [生]免疫缺陷

telltale /'telteɪl/ adj. 泄露内情的,报警的
myocardial /ˌmaɪəʊ'kɑːdiəl/ adj. [解]心肌的
infarction /ɪn'fɑːkʃən/ n. 梗死

herbicide /'hɜːbɪsaɪd/ n. 除草剂
pesticide /'pestɪsaɪd/ n. 杀虫剂

schizophrenia /ˌskɪzəʊˈfriːnɪə/ *n.* 精神分裂症

bases *for mental disorders such as Alzheimer disease and* schizophrenia? How does the immune system distinguish between self and nonself? What are the molecular mechanisms of short-term and long-term memory? The answers to such questions, which once seemed remote, have been partly uncovered and are likely to be more thoroughly revealed in the near future.

Task 1 **Find out the answers to the following questions and then compare your answers with a partner.**

1. What is biochemistry mainly concerned with? Why is it both a life science and chemical science?

2. What is the significance of understanding the essential life processes in biochemistry?

3. What are the biochemical differences between a human being and a chimpanzee?

4. What is the use of genetically engineered bacteria?

5. How does biochemistry research contribute to medical practice?

Part II Listening

Task 2 **You will hear 20 words or phrases which will be read three times. Write them down on the blanks and check with your partner after you finish.**

1. _____ 2. _____ 3. _____ 4. _____

5. _____ 6. _____ 7. _____ 8. _____

9. _____ 10. _____ 11. _____ 12. _____

13. _____ 14. _____ 15. _____ 16. _____

17. _____ 18. _____ 19. _____ 20. _____

Task 3 You are going to hear a passage which will be read three times. Take some notes while you are listening to the passage and then answer the following questions.

1. What does biochemistry study?

2. What life processes are chemical reactions involved in?

3. What does molecular biology study?

Part Ⅲ Oral Presentation and Discussion

Task 4 Read the following passage and make an oral presentation.

CRISPR Cancer Trial Success Paves the Way for Personalized Treatments

A small clinical trial has shown that researchers can use CRISPR gene editing to alter immune cells so that they will recognize mutated proteins specific to a person's tumors. Those cells can then be safely set loose in the body to find and destroy their target.

It is the first attempt to combine two hot areas in cancer research: gene editing to create personalized treatments, and engineering immune cells called T cells so as to better target tumors. The approach was tested in 16 people with solid tumors, including in the breast and colon.

"It is probably the most complicated therapy ever attempted in the clinic," says study co-author Antoni Ribas, a cancer researcher and physician at the University of California, Los Angeles. "We're trying to make an army out of a patient's own T cells."

The results were published in *Nature* and presented at the Society for Immunotherapy of Cancer meeting in Boston, Massachusetts on 10 November.

Tailored Treatments

Ribas and his colleagues began by sequencing DNA from blood samples and tumour biopsies, to look for mutations that are found in the tumour but not in the blood. This had to be done for each person in the trial. "The mutations are different in every cancer," says Ribas. "And although there are some shared mutations, they are the minority."

The researchers then used algorithms to predict which of the mutations were likely to be capable of provoking a response from T cells, a type of white blood cell that patrols the body looking for errant cells. "If [T cells] see something that looks not normal, they kill it," says Stephanie Mandl, chief scientific officer at PACT Pharma in South San Francisco, California, and a lead author on the study. "But in the patients we see in the clinic with cancer, at some point the immune system kind of lost the battle and the tumour grew."

After a series of analyses to confirm their findings, validate their predictions and design proteins called T-cell receptors that are capable of recognizing the tumour mutations, the researchers took blood samples from each participant and used CRISPR genome editing to insert the genes encoding these receptors into their T cells. Each participant then had to take medication to reduce the number of immune cells they produced, and the engineered cells were infused.

"This is a tremendously complicated manufacturing process," says Joseph Fraietta, who designs T-cell cancer therapies at the University of Pennsylvania in Philadelphia. In some cases, the entire procedure took more than one year.

Each of the 16 participants received engineered T cells with up to three different targets. Afterwards, the edited cells were found circulating in their blood, and were present in higher concentrations near tumors than non-edited cells had been prior to the treatment. One month after treatment, five of the participants experienced stable disease, meaning that their tumors had not grown. Only two people experienced side effects that were probably due to the activity of the edited T cells.

Although the efficacy of the treatment was low, the researchers used relatively small doses of T cells to establish the safety of the approach, says Ribas. "We just need to hit it stronger the next time," he says.

And as researchers develop ways to speed up the therapies' development, the engineered cells will spend less time being cultured outside of the body and could be more active when they are infused. "The technology will get better and better," says Fraietta.

A Solid Start

Engineered T cells—called CAR T cells—have been approved for the treatment of some blood and lymph cancers, but solid tumours have posed a particular challenge. CAR T cells are effective only against proteins that are expressed on the surface of tumour cells. Such proteins can be found across many blood and lymph cancers, which means there is no need to design new T-cell receptors for each person with cancer.

But common surface proteins have not been found in solid tumors, says Fraietta. And solid tumors provide physical barriers to T cells, which must circulate through the blood, travel to the tumour and then infiltrate it to kill the cancer cells. Tumour cells also sometimes suppress immune responses, both by releasing immune-suppressing chemical signals and by using up the local supply of nutrients to fuel their rapid growth.

"The environment around a tumour is like a sewer," says Fraietta. "T cells are rendered less functional as soon as they hit the site."

With this initial proof of concept in hand, Mandl and her colleagues hope to be able to engineer T cells not only to recognize cancer mutations, but also to be more active near the tumour. Mandl says there are several potential ways to toughen up T cells, for example by removing the receptors that respond to immuno-suppressive signals, or by tweaking their metabolism so that they can more easily find an energy source in the tumour environment.

Such elaborate designs could be feasible thanks to recent technological advances in using CRISPR to edit T cells, says Avery

Posey, who studies cell and gene therapies for cancer at the University of Pennsylvania. "It's become incredibly efficient," he says. "We'll see very sophisticated means of engineering immune cells within the next decade."

Task 5 **Theme-related discussion.**

Genetic engineering has made great achievements in biomedicine, modern agriculture, environmental pollution control, and the transformation of traditional biotechnology. For instance, scientists have used gene-editing tools to make personalized modifications to cancer patients' immune cells to target tumors better.

Please watch the MOOC, think about it, and discuss the following questions with your partner.

1. What are the applications of genetic engineering in modern medicine?

2. What are the major concerns about the use of genetic technologies in the health sector?

Part IV Word Formation

sack, bladder [英] 囊,膀胱

  cyst(o)- 囊,膀胱

    cystoscope /ˈsɪstəʊskəʊp/ n. 膀胱镜

    cystotomy /sɪsˈtɒtəmi/ n. 膀胱切开术

    nephrocystitis /ˌnefrəʊsɪsˈtaɪtɪs/ n. 肾膀胱炎

fiber [英] 纤维

  fibr(o)- [拉] 纤维

    fibrescope /ˈfaɪbəskəʊp/ n. 纤维内窥镜

    fibrillation /ˌfɪbrɪˈleɪʃən/ n. 纤维性颤动

    fibrinolysis /ˌfaɪbrɪˈnɒlɪsɪs/ n. 纤维蛋白溶解

blood [英] 血

  hemat(o)-,hem(o)- [希] 血

    hematology /ˌhiːməˈtɒlədʒi/ n. 血液学

    hematocyte /ˈhiːmətəʊsaɪt/ n. 血细胞

    hemotoxic /ˌhiːməʊˈtɒksɪk/ adj. 血中毒的

muscle [英] 肌肉

  my(o)- [希] 肌肉

    myoalbumin /ˌmaɪəʊæl'bjʊmɪn/ *n*. 肌清蛋白, 肌白蛋白

    myoatrophy /ˌmaɪəʊ'ætrəfi/ *n*. 肌萎缩

    myocardial /ˌmaɪəʊ'kɑːdiəl/ *adj*. 心肌的

under [英] 下, 低

  hyp(o)- [希] 在……之下, 亚, 不足

    hypodermic /ˌhaɪpəʊ'dɜːmɪk/ *adj*. 皮下的

    hypoadrenia /ˌhaɪpəʊə'driːniə/ *n*. 肾上腺功能减退

    hypocapnia /ˌhaɪpəʊ'kæpniə/ *n*. 低碳酸血（症）

    hypoliposis /ˌhaɪpəʊlɪ'pəʊsɪs/ *n*. 脂肪过少

bleeding [英] 出血

  -emia [希] 血症

    hypercythemia /ˌhaɪpəsaɪ'θiːmiə/ *n*. 红细胞增多症

    hyperalonemia /ˌhaɪpəæləʊ'niːmiə/ *n*. 血盐过多, 高盐血症

    pyrenemia /ˌpaɪrə'niːmiə/ *n*. 有核红细胞血症

    myxaemia /mɪk'siːmiə/ *n*. 粘蛋白血症

disease [英] 疾病

-ia [拉] 状态, 病名

    leukemia /ljuː'kiːmiə/ *n*. 白血病

    ataxia /ə'tæksiə/ *n*. 共济失调

    telangiectasia /təlˌændʒɪˌek'teɪʒiə/ *n*. 毛细血管扩张

Task 6 **Match each of the following terms with its definition.**

1	anemia	A	muscular strength
2	cystitis	B	the destruction or dissolution of red blood cells
3	myodynamia	C	deficiency in the amount of oxygen reaching body tissues
4	hypoxia	D	the formation of excessive fibrous tissue
5	fibrosis	E	a condition in which the concentration of red blood cells is too low
6	hemolysis	F	inflammation of the urinary bladder

Task 7 **Fill in the blanks with words or phrases given in the box. Change the form where necessary.**

hematocyte	hypothermia	cystoscope	myocardial infarction
hemoglobin	myocardium	leukemia	hemorrhagic shock
fibroma	hypodermic		

1. Most often, _____ is a cancer of the white blood cells, but some start in other blood cell types.

2. The _____ has a lens on the end that works like a telescope to magnify the inner surfaces of the urethra and bladder.

3. In humans, _____ is defined as a drop of core body temperature (or rectal temperature, in clinical practice) below 35 ℃.

4. _____ is a clinical syndrome resulting from decreased blood volume caused by blood loss, which leads to reduced cardiac output and organ perfusion.

5. The insulin can be taken up by diabetics by simple inhalation of the dispersed glassy particles instead of by _____ injection.

6. A blood cell, also called as _____, is a cell produced through hematopoiesis and is normally found in blood.

7. _____, commonly known as a heart attack, is the irreversible necrosis of heart muscle secondary to prolonged ischemia.

8. Your _____ level reflects the number of red blood cells in your body and how efficiently they carry oxygen to your cells.

9. _____ are noncancerous, which means they're typically not serious or life-threatening.

10. The _____ of the heart is the muscular middle layer of the heart that is sandwiched between the epicardium and endocardium.

Part V Fast Reading

From Guthrie to Genomes: The Continued Evolution of Newborn Screening

Introduction

Newborn screening (NBS) is one of the most valued public health programs in the US. Through NBS, approximately 15,000 newborns are identified annually with conditions for which screening, diagnosis, and effective treatments can be used early in life to significantly impact infant morbidity and mortality. Wilson and Jungner described the key features of disease screening in populations as:

"The central idea of early disease detection and treatment is essentially simple. However, the path to its successful achievement (on the one hand, bringing to treatment those with previously undetected disease; and, on the other, avoiding harm to those persons not in need of treatment) is far from simple though sometimes it may appear deceptively easy."

Two recent articles by Bick et al. and Watson et al. discussed the future of newborn screening and identified considerations and needs for the evolution of the newborn screening system as it tries to meet the growing demands to screen for more rare diseases and incorporate genomic technologies.

As NBS moves past 60 years of existence, there is great interest in how this successful public health program will continue to progress. Our understanding of the over 7000 known rare diseases has grown and the potential for use of genomic technologies at the population level has become more feasible leading to a heightened call for a newborn screening evolution. This has led to the development of both public and private programs that seek to expand newborn screening by assessing the clinical utility of next-generation sequencing in healthy newborns.

Faster Development of Therapies Will Likely Make It Appropriate to Screen for More Rare Diseases

A key criterion for a disease to be added to newborn screening is the availability of an effective treatment. Historically, meeting this measure has been one of the limiting factors in diseases being added to newborn screening panels. However, owing to programs like the Orphan Drug Act of 1983 and the Food and Drug Administration's Accelerated Approval Pathway, treatments and clinical trials for rare diseases have increased significantly. Currently, the FDA expects to receive 200 investigational new drug applications annually and anticipates soon approving 10 – 20 cell and gene therapies each year.

The addition of Spinal Muscular Atrophy (SMA) to the Health

and Human Services' Recommended Uniform Screening Panel (RUSP) is a recent success story illustrating the convergence of new life-changing therapies with newborn screening. The availability of innovative therapies for SMA, including gene therapy, enabled it to be added to the RUSP in 2018. The availability of these therapies, combined with the ability to multiplex screening for SMA with an existing molecular test, allowed for relatively rapid implementation throughout the country. Already, 92% of all babies born in U. S. states and territories are being screened for SMA, and this will soon reach 100%. SMA is likely the first of many diseases that will be added to newborn screening panels because of improved therapeutic strategies. CDC plays an important role in supporting newborn screening for all diseases on the RUSP, including SMA.

Throughout the history of newborn screening, addition of diseases to the RUSP has been guided by the ten principles for population screening developed by Wilson and Jungner. Both articles expand on the Wilson and Jungner principles to create possible criteria for prioritizing genes and diseases appropriate for public health newborn screening:

- Disease should be a significant health problem.
- Disease should be well categorized and understood.
- Treatment is available and accessible.
- Neither the test nor the treatment should add undue burden or harm to the population served.

As Bick, et al. and Watson, et al. point out, the rapid development of new therapies will greatly impact newborn screening programs as the number of candidate diseases for screening will very likely increase at a pace not sustainable by the current system. This gap might be closed by genomic sequencing technologies, which would allow for multiplexing multiple disease-causing genes with the ability to expand to additional genes relatively quickly.

Considerations for Incorporation of Genomic Technologies

Bick, et al. describe a potential newborn screening genomic sequencing protocol in which both gene and variant filters are applied to keep test sensitivity and specificity high. These filters would be derived from existing knowledge of the underlying genetics of the disease, which up to this point have predominantly been gleaned from White Non-Hispanic persons. This screening would be more likely to miss affected newborns of other races, increasing the already present health disparities among certain populations. However, if genomic-based screening were to expand to include variants of uncertain significance (as would likely be done in a mandated public health context), we risk a significant increase in false positive or uncertain screening results. In some cases, these types of results have been reported to cause psychological distress to families and may lead to the potential for increased costs to monitor asymptomatic, but screen positive infants. In addition, Bick et al. note:

Despite the great potential and flexibility of sequence-based testing, it is unlikely to replace current newborn screening. Many cases of congenital hypothyroidism do not have an identifiable molecular basis. Additionally, the analyte screen now in use has greater sensitivity and specificity for the disorders currently tested than genomic testing.

While genomic testing may not supplant the existing system for all current diseases, novel therapies are driving the introduction of new diseases where genome sequencing is likely to be used. Thus, the implications for exacerbating health disparities or causing psychological or financial harm must continue to be considered. Likewise, diversification of genomic research, such as in the All of Us Research Program, remains pivotal to equitable use of genomic sequencing in newborn screening.

Identified Challenges for the Future of Newborn Screening Programs

The successful evolution of newborn screening programs will require shifts, sometimes substantial, in public health infrastructure and resources with a continued eye towards health equity. Watson, et al. identify priority needs for systemic change:

• Redefined criteria for the targets and timing of newborn and child screening—be clear on the forms of the disease (e. g., infantile versus later-onset) that are the focus of screening and examine the potential for screening over the life course.

• Financing of the newborn screening system, including pilot programs for newborn screening state programs—continuous evaluation of funding for the entirety of the newborn screening system to ensure equitable and sustainable funding across the country.

• Building a national quality assurance infrastructure—develop standards for screening performance metrics and develop analytic tools that enhance disease detection.

• Promoting data and IT communications infrastructure—improve current newborn screening interoperability capacity and existing information systems.

• Fostering intra-government cooperation and communications—examine potential for central coordination that organizes federal agencies and intersects state newborn screening programs.

Both commentaries provide thoughtful examination of the ethical, communication, data management and transparency considerations as the public health newborn screening system looks to expand testing and treatment using genomic sequencing and new therapeutic technologies. These technologies hold great promise so long as the needs and concerns of all newborns and families remain at the center of deliberations.

Task 8 Read the passage and decide whether the statements are true or false. If it is true, write "T". If it is not, write "F".

1. Bick et al. and Watson et al. emphasized the importance of incorporating genomic technologies in future newborn screening technologies. ( )

2. A key criterion for a disease to be added to newborn screening is the availability of an effective treatment. ( )

3. SMA is likely the first of many diseases that will be added to newborn screening panels because of improved therapeutic strategies. ( )

4. Due to the great potential and flexibility of sequence-based testing, it is likely to replace current newborn screening. ( )

5. The successful evolution of newborn screening programs will require shifts in public health infrastructure and resources. ( )

Task 9 Please read the passage again and write a two-hundred-word synopsis.

Part Ⅵ Translation

Task 10 **Analyze the following sentences and then put them into Chinese.**

1. It uses the methods of chemistry, physics, molecular biology and immunology to study the structure and behavior of the complex molecules found in biological material and the ways those molecules interact to form cells, tissues and whole organism.

_____

_____

2. The researchers then used algorithms to predict which of the mutations were likely to be capable of provoking a response from T cells, a type of white blood cell that patrols the body looking for errant cells.

_____

_____

3. However, if genomic-based screening were to expand to include variants of uncertain significance (as would likely be done in a mandated public health context), we risk a significant increase in false positive or uncertain screening results.

_____

_____

医学翻译技巧

语 态

医学论文英文摘要采用何种语态,既要考虑摘要的特点,又要满足表达的需要。在英文摘要中,过去一般主张少用第一人称和主动语态,多用第三人称和被动语态。比如描述研究意图时很少用"我"或"我们",而是用"本文""本研究""本项实验"或"作者"等,即"This paper ...""This study ...""This research""The author(s)..."等等。

例 1　Based on a brief description of the structure and functions of HIF, this article discusses the relationship between inflammation, tumor and HIF.
本文在扼要叙述缺氧诱导因子 HIF 结构与功能的基础上,探讨 HIF 与炎症和肿瘤的关系。

再如叙述某一执行过程,可不必以作者为主语,而以事实本身为主语。

例 2　ASICs currents evoked by extracellular solutions of various pH values were recorded and analyzed in acute isolated rat DRG neurons by using whole-cell patch clamp technique.

应用全细胞膜片钳技术,在急性分散的成年大鼠 DRG 细胞上记录并分析由不同浓度 H⁺(降低 pH 值)诱发的 ASICs 电流。

又如做结论时,往往将第一人称的主动语态改为第三人称的被动语态,比如将"We suggest that …"写成"It is suggested that …"或"The facts suggest that …";将"We conclude that …"写成"It is concluded that …"。

例 3　It is concluded that DIC is a deteriorative factor in the pathogenesis of shock.
　　　DIC 是休克发病的恶化因子。

目前,越来越多的学者认为,在英文摘要及篇章写作中主动语态的使用可使表达更为有力,更简洁精确。

例 4　We developed a strategy to search MEDLINE to identify relevant articles. We selected search terms to capture categories of conditions(e. g, developmental disabilities, obesity), screening tests, specific interventions, and primary care.
　　　我们应用一个搜索 MEDLINE 的方法来确定相关的文章,选择一些搜索词条以采集疾病(例如:发育障碍、肥胖)、筛查检测、具体的干预措施以及初级保健等类别。

有时在同一段落中,也会依据篇章衔接性的需求同时使用主动语态与被动语态。

例 5　The Institutional Review Board approved this retrospective study from archival material from patients consenting to the use of medical records for research purposes. A retrospective review of contrast-enhanced abdominal CT scans in 45 patients (mean age, 59.5 years; range, 24—84 years) was performed.
　　　机构审查委员会批准了这项对患者病历的回顾性研究,并征得了患者同意。研究者对这 45 位接受腹部增强 CT 扫描的患者(平均年龄:59.5 岁;年龄范围:24～84 岁)开展了回顾性研究。

语态应依据是否需要提及或强调动作的发出者来确定,上例中第一句话是要强调本研究的合法性,因此采用了主动语态,点明批准本项研究的机构。而在后面的语句中,无须机械地强调回顾性研究实施的主体,故采用了被动语态。

从语法和篇章角度来看,主动语态与被动语态的使用各有特色,在论文中选用哪种语态应依实际需要与所投刊物用稿要求而定。有的刊物,如美国的《科学》杂志明确规定要多使用主动语态,以便于读者理解。此外,原来医学论文摘要的首句多用第三人称"This paper …"等开头,现在则倾向于采用更简洁的被动语态或原形动词开头,例如:"To describe …""To study …""To investigate …""To assess …""To determine …"等。

1. 这篇文章表明 B 超对宫外孕的早期诊断及鉴别有重要的应用价值。

2. 我们的研究表明，并非所有的运动都与乳腺癌有关。

3. 目的：探讨腺性膀胱炎临床特征和治疗效果。

4. 年龄、家庭收入、最高学历、婚姻状况、在家中使用最多的语言以及被访者能用以交谈的语言也是考察的因素。

5. 危重疾病常伴有高皮质醇血症。

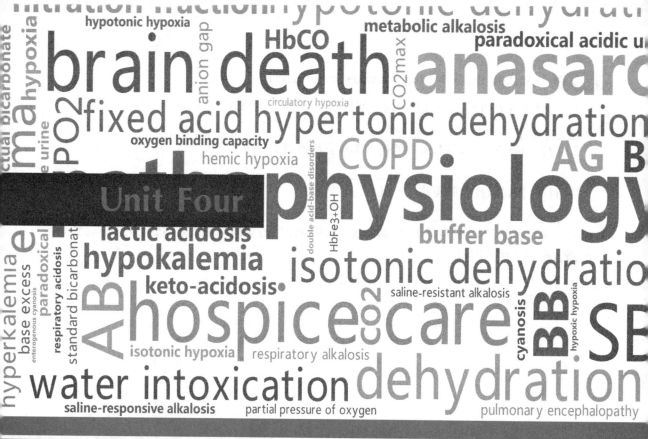

Pathology

✓课文音频
✓听力音频
✓在线课程
✓课件申请

An Introduction to Pathology

Pathology is the scientific study of disease. In clinical practice and medical education, pathology also has a wider meaning: pathology constitutes a large body of scientific knowledge, ideas and investigative methods essential for the understanding and practice of modern medicine.

pathology /pəˈθɒlədʒi/ n. 病理学,病理;病状

Pathology is not synonymous with the morphology of diseased tissues; this is an outmoded perception. Pathology includes knowledge and understanding of the functional and structural changes in disease, from the molecular level to the effects on the individual.

synonymous /sɪˈnɒnɪməs/ adj. 同义的
morphology /mɔːˈfɒlədʒi/ n. 形态学
outmoded /aʊtˈməʊdɪd/ adj. 过时的

Pathology is continually subject to change, revision and expansion as the application of new scientific methods illuminates our knowledge of disease.

The ultimate goal of pathology is the identification of the causes of disease, a fundamental objective that leads the way to disease prevention.

The Scope of Pathology

Pathology is the foundation of medical science and practice. Without pathology, the practice of medicine would be reduced to myths and folklore.

Clinical and experimental pathology

Scientific knowledge about human diseases is derived from observations on patients or, by analogy, from experimental studies on animals and cell culture. The greatest contribution comes from the study in depth of tissue and body fluids from patients.

analogy /əˈnælədʒi/ n. 类比,比拟

Clinical pathology

Clinical medicine is based on a longitudinal approach to patient's illness—the patient's history, the examination and investigation and the treatment. Clinical pathology is more concerned with a cross-sectional analysis at the level of the disease itself, studied in depth—the cause and mechanism of the disease, and the effects of the disease upon the various organs and systems of the body. These two perspectives are complementary and inseparable. Clinical medicine cannot be practiced without an understanding of pathology; pathology is meaningless if it is **bereft** of clinical implications.

Experimental pathology

Experimental pathology is the observation of the effects of manipulations on experimental systems such as animal models of disease or cell cultures. Fortunately, advances in cell culture technology have reduced the usage of laboratory animals in medical research and experimental pathology. However, it is extremely difficult to reproduce in cell cultures the physiological **milieu** that prevails in the intact human body.

Subdivisions of pathology

Pathology is a vast subject with many **ramifications**. In practice, however, it can be split into major subdivisions:

- **Histopathology**: the investigation and diagnosis of disease from the examination of tissues.
- **Cytopathology**: the investigation and diagnosis of disease from the examination of isolated cells.
- **Haematology**: the study of disorders of the **cellular** and **coagulable** components of blood.
- **Microbiology**: the study of infectious diseases and the organisms responsible for them.
- **Immunology**: the study of the specific defence mechanism of the body.
- **Chemical pathology**: the study and diagnosis of disease from the chemical changes in tissues and fluids.
- **Genetics**: the study of abnormal **chromosomes** and genes.
- **Toxicology**: the study of the effects of known or suspected poisons.

---

bereft /bɪˈreft/ *adj.* 丧失……的;被剥夺……的

milieu /miˈljuː/ *n.* 环境

ramification /ˌræmɪfɪˈkeɪʃən/ *n.* 分叉,分支;衍生物

histopathology /ˌhɪstəʊpəˈθɒlədʒi/ *n.* 组织病理学

cytopathology /ˌsaɪtəʊpəˈθɒlədʒi/ *n.* 细胞病理学

haematology /ˌhiːməˈtɒlədʒi/ *n.* 血液学,血液病学

cellular /ˈseljʊlə/ *adj.* 细胞的,细胞质的;细胞状的

coagulable /kəʊˈægjʊləbl/ *adj.* 可凝结的

chromosome /ˈkrəʊməsəʊm/ *n.* 染色体

toxicology /ˌtɒksɪˈkɒlədʒi/ *n.* 毒理学,毒物学

• Forensic pathology: the application of pathology to legal purposes (e. g. investigation of death in suspicious circumstances).

These subdivisions are more important professionally (because each requires its own team of specialists) than educationally. The subject must be taught and learnt in an integrated manner, for the body and its disease make no distinction between these conventional subdivisions.

General and Systematic Pathology

Pathology is best taught and learnt in two stages:

• General pathology: the mechanisms and characteristics of the principal types of disease process (e. g. congenital versus acquired diseases, inflammation, tumors, degenerations).

• Systematic pathology: the descriptions of specific diseases as they affect individual organs or organ systems (e. g. appendicitis, lung cancer, atheroma).

General pathology

General pathology is our current understanding of the causation, mechanisms and characteristics of the major categories of disease.

It is essential that the principles of general pathology are understood before an attempt is made to study systematic pathology. General pathology is the foundation of knowledge that has to be laid down before one can begin to study the systematic pathology of specific diseases.

Systematic pathology

Systematic pathology is our current knowledge of specific diseases as they affect individual organs or systems. ("Systematic" should not be confused with "systemic" in this context. Systemic pathology would be characteristic of a disease that pervaded *all* body systems. Each specific disease can usually be attributed to the operation of one or more categories of causation and mechanism featuring in general pathology. Thus, acute appendicitis is acute inflammation affecting the appendix; carcinoma of the lung is the result of

forensic /fəˈrensɪk/ *adj.* 法医的，应用法律程序的

congenital /kɒnˈdʒenɪtl/ *adj.*（指疾病等）生来的，先天的
inflammation /ˌɪnfləˈmeɪʃən/ *n.* 红肿，炎症
tumor /ˈtjuːmə/ *n.* 肿块，肿瘤
degeneration /dɪˌdʒenəˈreɪʃ(ə)n/ *n.* 退化；变性
appendicitis /əˌpendɪˈsaɪtɪs/ *n.* 阑尾炎
atheroma /ˌæθəˈrəʊmə/ *n.*（*pl.* atheromas, atheromata）粥样斑

systemic /sɪsˈtemɪk/ *adj.* 全身的

carcinoma /ˌkɑːsɪˈnəʊmə/ *n.*（*pl.* carcinomas, carcinomata）癌

carcinogenesis acting upon cells in the lung, and the behavior of the cancerous cells thus formed follows the pattern established for malignant tumors; and so on.

Task 1 **Find out the answers to the following questions and then compare your answers with a partner.**

1. What is the ultimate goal of pathology?

2. How can the relationship between clinical medicine and pathology be understood?

3. What is the aim of experimental pathology?

4. Is it true that one should learn the systematic pathology of specific diseases before one begins to study general pathology?

5. Is systematic pathology the same as systemic pathology? And why?

Part II Listening

Task 2 **You will hear 20 words or phrases which will be read three times. Write them down on the blanks and check with your partner after you finish.**

1. _____	2. _____	3. _____	4. _____
5. _____	6. _____	7. _____	8. _____
9. _____	10. _____	11. _____	12. _____
13. _____	14. _____	15. _____	16. _____
17. _____	18. _____	19. _____	20. _____

Task 3 **You are going to hear a passage which will be read three times. Take some notes while you are listening to the passage and then answer the following questions.**

1. What does pathology provide to patients and clinicians?

_____

2. How important is a pathologist in medical care?

_____

3. What modalities do pathologists use to determine the presence of disease?

Part Ⅲ　Oral Presentation and Discussion

Task 4 Read the following passage and make an oral presentation.

Will Animal Test be Phased Out?

The Food and Drug Administration commits to exploring alternative methods to replace laboratory animals in developing new drugs and products.

The future of drug development might be animal-free—or, at least, involve far fewer animals than is currently the norm. Last June, the US Food and Drug Administration (FDA) set out proposals for the New Alternative Methods Program that will focus on replacing, reducing and refining the use of laboratory animals through the adoption of cutting-edge alternative methods. The aim is to produce findings that are more relevant to humans, streamline product development and reduce costs.

The shift, which has been years in the making, would be undertaken across all of the FDA's centres, including ones that oversee the approval of new pharmaceuticals, medical devices, veterinary medicines, cosmetics and more. FDA scientists are conducting their own research in service of this goal and are collaborating extensively with colleagues in industry, academia and other sectors. Any methods eventually adopted in place of research involving animals would be rigorously vetted and "fully validated and based on the best science", says Namandjé Bumpus, chief scientist at the FDA. Bumpus and her colleagues have not received any pushback from researchers about making this shift, she adds, or heard any concerns from the scientific community about cutting back on the use of animals.

Although there is no set timeline, FDA officials say the programme is a priority. It would be funded ＄5 million it has requested as part of its 2023 budget to develop a "comprehensive strategy" on alternative testing methods. According to Paul Locke, an environmental-health scientist and lawyer at Johns Hopkins University in Baltimore, Maryland, who specializes in alternatives to animal testing, the FDA is taking a necessary step towards ensuring that the US government stays up to speed with the latest science. "I'm really excited about what the FDA's doing here," he says. "They've put a stake in the ground and said, 'Hey, we want to be there using these tools, they're consistent with our mission and they're consistent with what twenty-first-century science looks like.'"

Biomedical Advances Fuel Alternatives

Animal-based testing has been the gold standard for research for decades, and it remains an important requirement for establishing the safety and efficacy of products being brought to market today. But key differences exist between humans and the rodents, rabbits, non-human primates and other animals that researchers depend on for testing, and as biomedical understanding has advanced, scientists have begun to come up against the limitations of using other species as proxies for humans. "A mouse or a rat doesn't always handle or process medicines and chemicals in the same way humans do," Bumpus says. "Developing more in vitro systems that are based on human cells, human tissues and human models could, in some instances, be more predictive."

The FDA's interest in moving towards new approaches also reflects the current thinking of the biomedical community at large. In 2014, the United Kingdom, for example, announced plans to reduce the use of animal tests in scientific research, aiming to replace those tests with "scientifically valid alternatives" where possible. In 2021, the European Parliament voted in favour of plans to phase out animal testing in research.

"A key for bringing about change is to do so among the multiple major regulatory agencies," says David Strauss, director of the FDA's Division of Applied Regulatory Science. "Drug-development programmes are global, and companies want to market their products in many countries around the world."

That sentiment is echoed by Bumpus. "There's a lot of energy around this across the globe," she adds.

Animal-rights advocates have been calling for an end to animal testing for years; now, methods being developed in labs around the world have made this a realistic possibility for the future. "We think we're at a potential tipping point," says Strauss. The technologies include, for example, induced pluripotent stem cells—cells that scientists program to have the potential to turn into any cell type found in the body—and "organs-on-a-chip", which are small devices containing living human tissues that mimic an organ, organ system or even an entire body. Developments in artificial intelligence and machine learning are also allowing scientists to harness existing data to build computer models that can make predictions about a new drug's safety and efficacy.

More Funding Needed

In addition to being more relevant to humans, says Locke, once these types of technology are qualified and validated for specific uses, they will probably be faster and cheaper than using animals, allowing products to be brought to market more rapidly and efficiently. These are still early days, however, and so far, the FDA has only a handful of successful animal-testing-replacement stories it can point to.

Funding for developing and validating alternative methods is also an issue, Locke adds—both internally at the FDA, and externally for scientists whose labs depend on federal funds to pioneer new approaches. The FDA is not primarily a funding agency, and the US National Institutes of Health, which is the largest public funder of biomedical research in the world, currently has no programme dedicated to developing alternatives to animal testing. "If we had a legitimate funding programme to push these technologies forward, it would accelerate their progress greatly," Locke points out.

For now, despite the promising alternatives to animal testing, federal regulators have approved only a few cutting-edge methods, and such techniques will not completely replace animal testing any time soon. But they do hold great promise, Locke says, especially if other government agencies and countries join the FDA in its effort.

"There's a lot of moving pieces here," he says. "The FDA has started the ball rolling, but we need more work to make sure we can use these new methodologies appropriately."

Task 5 Theme-related discussion.

Animal testing, also known as animal experiment or research, is the use of non-human animals in experiments that aims to control the variables that affect biological systems and the behaviors under study. Whether experiments can be conducted with animals has aroused heated discussion.

Please watch the MOOC, think about it, and discuss the following questions with your partner.

1. What are the main reasons to support or oppose animal testing?

2. What are the possible alternatives to animal testing in the future?

Part Ⅳ Word Formation

disease [英] 疾病

    path(o)- [希] 病理,疾病

        pathography /pəˈθɒɡrəfi/ *n*. 病情记录

        pathogenesis /ˌpæθəˈdʒenɪsɪs/ *n*. 发病机制

        pathomorphism /ˌpæθəˈmɔːfɪzəm/ *n*. 病理形态学

color [英] 颜色

    chrom(o)- [希] 色

        chromoblast /ˈkrəʊməblɑːst/ *n*. 成色素细胞

        chromosomal /ˌkrəʊməˈsəʊməl/ *adj*. 染色体的

        chromophototherapy /ˌkrəʊməˌfəʊtəʊˈθerəpi/ *n*. 色光疗法

cell [英] 细胞

    -cyte [希] 细胞

        pneumocyte /ˈnjuːməsaɪt/ *n*. 肺细胞

        cardiocyte /ˈkɑːdiəʊsaɪt/ *n*. 心肌细胞

cytology /saɪˈtɒlədʒi/ n. 细胞学

poison [英] 毒素, 毒

  tox(o)- [希] 毒, 毒素

    toxoid /ˈtɒksɒɪd/ n. 类毒素

    toxinemia /ˌtɒksɪˈniːmiə/ n. 毒血症

    toxuria /tɒkˈsjuːriə/ n. 尿毒症

tumor [英] 瘤

  -oma 瘤病

    nephroma /neˈfrəʊmə/ n. 肾瘤

    neuroma /njʊˈrəʊmə/ n. 神经瘤

    myoma /maɪˈəʊmə/ n. 肌瘤

producing [英] 产生

  -genesis [希] 产生, 生成

    myelogenesis /ˌmaɪələʊˈdʒenɪsɪs/ n. 髓发生

    pathogenesis /ˌpæθəˈdʒenɪsɪs/ n. 发病机制

    dentinogenesis /ˌdentɪnəʊˈdʒenɪsɪs/ n. 牙本质发生

spinal membrane [英] 脊髓膜

  mening(o)- [希] 脑膜, 脊髓膜

    meningorrhagia /məˌnɪŋgəʊˈreɪdʒiə/ n. 脑膜出血

    meningocyte /məˈnɪŋgəsaɪt/ n. 脑膜细胞

    meningoma /ˌmenɪnˈgəʊmə/ n. 脑膜瘤

Task 6 **Match each of the following terms with its definition.**

1	meninges	A	a type of cancer
2	chromosome	B	a white blood cell
3	carcinoma	C	the three fibrous membranes that cover and protect the brain and spinal cord
4	pathogenicity	D	a condition in which the blood contains bacterial products
5	leukocyte	E	the ability to cause a disease
6	toxemia	F	a thread-like structure made of DNA and proteins present in the nucleus of cells

Task 7 **Fill in the blanks with words or phrases given in the box. Change the form where necessary.**

congenital	chromatin	pathogenesis	pathogen
meningitis	toxic	pneumocyte	coagulate
pathophysiology	chromosomal		

1. _____ refers to a mixture of DNA and proteins that form the chromosomes found in the cells of humans and other higher organisms.

2. A microbe that is capable of causing disease is referred to as a _____ , while the organism being infected is called a host.

3. The cells that line the alveoli and comprise of the majority of the inner surface of the lungs are called alveolar cells, or _____ .

4. _____ seeks to reveal the physiologic responses of an organism to disruptions in its internal or external environment.

5. Chromosome deletion, duplication, inversion, and translation are known to cause different kinds of genetic and _____ mutation diseases.

6. Blood clotting, or _____ , is an important process that prevents excessive bleeding when a blood vessel is injured.

7. _____ refers to the development or evolution of a disease, from the initial stimulus to the ultimate expression of the manifestations of the disease.

8. An estimated 240 000 newborns die worldwide within 28 days of birth every year due to disorders.

9. Spinal _____ is an infection that causes inflammation of fluid and tissues surrounding the brain and spinal cord.

10. Chemical hazards and _____ substances pose a wide range of health hazards such as irritation and physical hazards such as flammability.

Part V Fast Reading

Types of Breast Cancer

The type of breast cancer you have helps determine the best approach to treating the disease. Get the facts on types of breast cancer and how they differ.

Your doctor suspects that you have breast cancer. To confirm the diagnosis, a pathologist analyzes a tissue sample taken from the lump or suspicious area in your breast. This will tell if you have cancer or some other, benign condition. If the biopsy does show cancer, the results provide your doctor with information about the type of breast cancer and help determine treatment options.

The biopsy results appear on a pathology report, which provides detailed information including the type of breast cancer, if it's invasive or noninvasive, the tumor grade—how closely the cancer cells resemble normal tissue—if the cancer is sensitive to hormonal therapies and if it has too much of a protein called HER-2.

Sophisticated lab tests can also analyze breast cancer tissue for molecular and genetic features of breast cancer cells. Understanding all these aspects of a cancer helps your doctor tailor your treatment plan.

Common Types of Breast Cancer

The most common types of breast cancer begin either in your breast's milk ducts (ductal carcinoma) or in the milk-producing glands (lobular carcinoma). The point of origin is determined by the appearance of the cancer cells under a microscope.

In situ breast cancer

In situ (noninvasive) breast cancer refers to cancer in which the cells have remained within their place of origin—they haven't spread to breast tissue around the duct or lobule. The most common type of noninvasive breast cancer is ductal carcinoma in situ, which is confined to the lining of the milk ducts. The abnormal cells haven't spread through the duct walls into surrounding breast tissue. With appropriate treatment, DCIS has an excellent prognosis.

Invasive breast cancer

Invasive (infiltrating) breast cancers spread outside the membrane that lines a duct or lobule, invading the surrounding tissues. The cancer cells can then travel to other parts of your body, such as the lymph nodes.

Invasive ductal carcinoma (IDC)

IDC accounts for about 70 percent of all breast cancers. The cancer cells form in the lining of your milk duct, then break through the ductal wall and invade nearby breast tissue. The cancer cells may remain localized—staying near the site of origin—or spread (metastasize) throughout your body, carried by your bloodstream or lymphatic system.

Invasive lobular carcinoma (ILC)

ILC, this type of breast cancer invades in a similar way, starting in the milk-producing lobules and then breaking into the surrounding breast tissue. ILC can also spread to more distant parts of your body. With this type of cancer, you typically won't feel a distinct, firm lump but rather a fullness or area of thickening.

Less Common Types of Breast Cancer

Not all types of breast cancer begin in a duct or lobule. Less common types of breast cancer may arise from the breast's supporting tissue, including the fibrous connective tissue, blood vessels and lymphatic system. In addition, some tumors don't actually begin in the breast but represent a different type of cancer that has spread (metastasized) from another part of the body, such as the lymphatic system (non-Hodgkin's lymphoma), skin (melanoma), colon or lungs. These are not called breast cancer but are referred to as cancer from where it started, now metastatic to the breast.

Unusual types of breast cancer include inflammatory breast cancer, phyllodes tumor, angiosarcoma, osteosarcoma, metaplastic breast cancer, adenoid cystic carcinoma and Paget's disease of the breast. There are also rare subtypes of invasive ductal carcinoma—tubular, mucinous, medullary and papillary.

Tumor grade

If the cancer is an invasive type, the pathologist assigns it a grade. The grade is based on how closely cells in the sample tissue resemble normal breast tissue under the microscope. The grading information, along with the cell type, helps your doctor determine treatment options.

Breast cancers are graded on a 1 to 3 scale:

Grade 1: The cells still look fairly normal (well differentiated).

Grade 2: The cells are somewhat abnormal (moderately differentiated).

Grade 3: The cells have lost their proper structure and function (poorly differentiated).

The pathologist determines the grade by looking at the size and shape of both the cell and its nucleus and counting how many cells are in the process of dividing. A higher grade suggests a faster growing cancer that's more likely to spread.

Hormone receptor status

Breast cancers are tested for the presence of estrogen and progesterone receptors. A receptor is a protein on the outside of a cell that can attach to specific chemicals, hormones or drugs traveling through the bloodstream.

Normal breast cells and some breast cancer cells have receptors that bind to the female hormones estrogen and progesterone. The hormones signal the cells to increase or "turn on" cell growth.

Breast cancers can be hormone receptor (HR) positive or HR negative. Tumors found to be HR positive are further categorized as estrogen receptor positive (ER positive) or progesterone receptor positive (PR positive). With ER positive or PR positive breast cancer, hormone-blocking medications, such as tamoxifen, slow the cancer's growth. Hormone receptor positive cancers typically grow more slowly than do HR negative cancers.

HER-2 status

Knowing if a cancer has too many copies of the HER-2 gene also influences treatment decisions. This gene drives production of the growth-promoting HER-2 protein. About one out of every five breast cancers is HER-2 positive, meaning these cancers have greater than normal amounts of the HER-2 protein. These cancers tend to grow and spread more aggressively than do other cancers.

Two sophisticated lab tests can detect HER-2 in cancer cells:

Immunohistochemistry. Special antibodies that attach to HER-2 protein are applied to the tissue sample, and cells change color if too many HER-2 protein receptors are present.

Fluorescent in situ hybridization (FISH). Fluorescent pieces of DNA find extra copies of the HER-2 gene. Chromogenic in situ hybridization is a similar technique.

Some laboratories use FISH only, since many breast cancer specialists believe this test is more accurate than is the immunohistochemistry test.

HER-2 positive breast cancers can be treated with drugs that specifically target the HER-2 protein, such as trastuzumab (Herceptin) and lapatinib (Tykerb).

Breast cancers that are HER-2 negative and also lack receptors for estrogen and progesterone are referred to as "triple negative". This form of the disease tends to be aggressive and may respond better to different treatments. It appears to be more common in young black and Hispanic women.

Emerging Ways to Classify Breast Cancer

The goal of much current breast cancer research is to understand the characteristics of cells in individual tumors. By applying the latest in molecular technology, researchers can identify genes associated with breast cancer and measure their activity in tissue samples. Tools called microarray analysis and reverse transcriptase-polymerase chain reaction (RT-PCR) are used to study patterns of behavior, or expression, of large numbers of genes in breast tissue samples. The researchers can then identify a set of genes whose activity provides information about a cancer, such as the likelihood of recurrence. These tests, known as genetic profiling or gene-expression profiling, have so far been used only for a minority of breast cancers.

Some researchers have proposed a new way to classify breast cancers based on molecular features rather than on the cancer's appearance under a microscope. These types include:

Luminal A and luminal B. The genetic activity of these cancers is similar to that of normal lumen cells—those that line the breast ducts and glands. Luminal cancers are estrogen receptor positive and usually grow slowly.

HER-2. These cancers have extra amounts of HER-2 protein and extra copies of the gene. They tend to grow quickly but respond well to treatment with Herceptin.

Basal. Basal breast cancers contain normal amounts of HER-2 and lack estrogen and progesterone receptors. This type of cancer grows rapidly.

Most doctors still use the traditional categories when talking about types of breast cancer. But they draw on the latest research about breast cancer features to determine the best course of treatment.

Task 8 **Read the passage and decide whether the statements are true or false. If it is true, write "T". If it is not, write "F".**

1. The most common types of breast cancer begin both in your breast's milk ducts (ductal carcinoma) and in the milk-producing glands (lobular carcinoma). (   )

2. A cancer in which the cells haven't spread to breast tissue around the duct or lobule is called invasive breast cancer. ( )

3. All types of breast cancer don't begin in a duct or lobule. ( )

4. Normal breast cells and some breast cancer cells have receptors that bind to the female hormones estrogen and progesterone. ( )

5. Most doctors have given up using the traditional categories when talking about types of breast cancer. ( )

Task 9 **Please read the passage again and write a two-hundred-word synopsis.**

Part VI Translation

Task 10 **Analyze the following sentences and then put them into Chinese.**

1. Pathology includes knowledge and understanding of the functional and structural changes in disease, from the molecular level to the effects on the individual.

_____

_____

2. Clinical pathology is more concerned with a cross-sectional analysis at the level of the disease itself, studied in depth—the cause and mechanism of the disease, and the effects of the disease upon the various organs and systems of the body.

_____

_____

3. Each specific disease can usually be attributed to the operation of one or more categories of causation and mechanism featuring in general pathology.

_____

_____

医学翻译技巧

名词化结构

科技语体具有科学性、准确性和抽象性三个特点。科技语体的抽象性主要体现在大量而准确地使用抽象名词这一语言手段上,名词化结构就是其代表,即在通用语体中用动词、形容词等词充当某种语法成分,而在科技语体中往往转为动词的名词形式来表达。这种结构往往用来表达最重要的信息内容,并使得科技文章的句子变长,信息结构变得复杂难懂。

例1 病人的病情开始好转后接着复发,是这种病的常见信号。

译文1 After the patient's condition began to <u>improve</u>, it <u>relapsed</u>, which is a common signal of this event.

译文2 *Relapse* following *initial improvement* <u>is</u> a common signal of this event.

例2 抑制菌群的某一部分,无疑会使其他细菌增殖。

译文1 To suppress a portion of the microflora inevitably makes other organisms be proliferated.

译文2 *The suppression of* a portion of the microflora inevitably <u>results in</u> the *proliferation of* other organisms.

以上两个例句,译文1显然比译文2容易理解。而译文2显得更简洁、客观,逻辑更加准确严密。

例3 生物化学<u>是</u>在细胞和分子水平上<u>运用</u>化学<u>研究</u>生物过程的一门学科。
　　　Biochemistry is <u>the application of</u> chemistry to <u>the study of</u> biological processes at the cellular and molecular level.

"运用化学研究生物……"是本句话的重要内容,用名词化结构表达既准确简洁,结构又严密。

例4 如果不懂得病理学,临床医学就无从开展。

译文1 Clinical medicine cannot be practiced if we do not understand pathology.

译文2 Clinical medicine cannot be practiced without an understanding of pathology.

译文2的表达比译文1显得更加客观。

Task 11 Translate the following sentences into English.

1. 病理学的最终目的在于确定疾病的原因,从而达到预防疾病的基本目的。

2. 病理学对理解现代医学及医学实践至关重要。

3. 衰老是一种正常的生理过程,伴有进行性改变肌体平衡适应性应答。

4. DNA 的重要性在于它能够控制细胞内蛋白质的形成。

5. 致病微生物侵入人体可引发严重疾病。

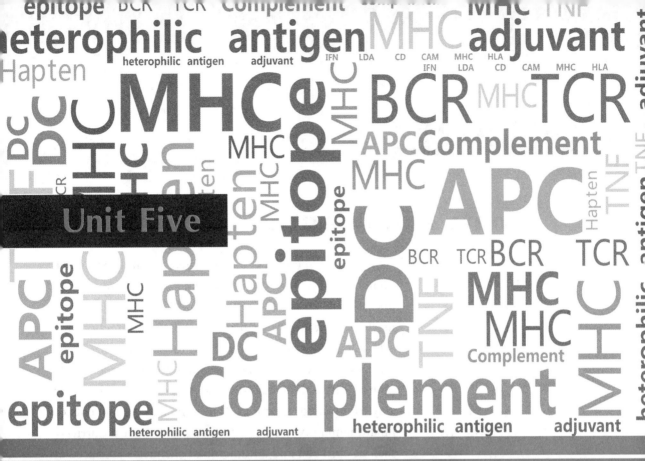

Unit Five

Immunology

✓课文音频
✓听力音频
✓在线课程
✓课件申请

Innate and Adaptive Immunity

innate immunity 固有免疫

microbe /ˈmaɪkrəʊb/ *n.* 微生物

barrier /ˈbæriə/ *n.* 障碍物，屏障

phagocytic /ˌfægəʊˈsɪtɪk/ *adj.* 噬菌细胞的，吞噬细胞的

neutrophil /ˈnjuːtrəʊfɪl/ *n.* 嗜中性粒细胞

dendritic /denˈdrɪtɪk/ *adj.* 树枝状的

cytokine /ˈsaɪtəʊkaɪn/ *n.* 细胞因子

magnitude /ˈmægnɪtjuːd/ *n.* 大小，规模；数量

exquisite /ɪkˈskwɪzɪt/ *adj.* 精致的；强烈的

Innate immunity（also called natural or native immunity）provides the early line of defense against microbes. It consists of cellular and biochemical defense mechanisms that are in place even before infection and are poised to respond rapidly to infections. These mechanisms react to microbes and to the products of injured cells, and they respond in essentially the same way to repeated infections. The principal components of innate immunity are（1）physical and chemical barriers, such as epithelia and antimicrobial chemicals produced at epithelial surfaces;（2）phagocytic cells（neutrophils, macrophages）, dendritic cells, and natural killer（NK）cells;（3）blood proteins, including members of the complement system and other mediators of inflammation; and（4）proteins called cytokines that regulate and coordinate many of the activities of the cells of innate immunity. The mechanisms of innate immunity are specific for structures that are common to groups of related microbes and may not distinguish fine differences between microbes.

In contrast to innate immunity, there are other immune responses that are stimulated by exposure to infectious agents and increase in magnitude and defensive capabilities with each successive exposure to a particular microbe. Because this form of immunity develops as a response to infection and adapts to the infection, it is called adaptive immunity. The defining characteristics of adaptive immunity are exquisite specificity for distinct molecules and an ability to "remember" and respond more vigorously to repeated exposures to the same microbe. The adaptive immune system is able to recognize and react to a large number of microbial and nonmicrobial substances. In addition, it has an extraordinary capacity to distinguish between different, even closely related, microbes and molecules, and for this reason it is also called specific immunity. It is also sometimes called acquired immunity, to emphasize that potent protective responses are "acquired" by experience. The main components of adaptive immunity are cells called lymphocytes and their secreted products, such as antibodies. Foreign substances that induce specific immune responses or are recognized by lymphocytes or antibodies are called antigens.

Mechanisms for defending the host against microbes are present in some form in all multicellular organisms. These mechanisms constitute innate immunity. The more specialized defense mechanisms that constitute adaptive immunity are found in vertebrates only. Two functionally similar but molecularly distinct adaptive immune systems developed at different times in evolution. About 500 million years ago, jawless fish, such as lampreys and hagfish, developed a unique immune system containing diverse lymphocyte-like cells that may function like lymphocytes in more advanced species and even responded to immunization. The antigen receptors on these cells were variable leucine-rich receptors that were capable of recognizing many antigens but were distinct from the antibodies and T cell receptors that appeared later in evolution. Most of the components of the adaptive immune system, including lymphocytes with highly diverse antigen receptors, antibodies, and specialized lymphoid tissues, evolved coordinately within a short time in jawed vertebrates (e. g., sharks), about 360 million years ago. The immune system has also become increasingly specialized with evolution.

Innate and adaptive immune responses are components of an integrated system of host defense in which numerous cells and molecules function cooperatively. The mechanisms of innate immunity provide effective initial defense against

potent /'pəʊtnt/ adj. 强有力的，有效的

lymphocyte /'lɪmfəsaɪt/ n. 淋巴细胞

antigen /'æntɪdʒən/ n. 抗原

lamprey /'læmpri/ n. 八目鳗，七鳃鳗
hagfish /'hægfɪʃ/ n. 蒲氏黏盲鳗
immunization /ˌɪmjuːnaɪ'zeɪʃən/ n. 免疫
leucine /'ljuːsiːn/ n. 亮氨酸，白氨酸

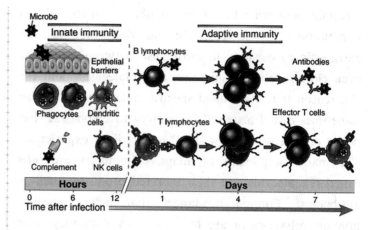

Microbe

Innate immunity   Adaptive immunity

Epithelial barriers   B lymphocytes   Antibodies

Phagocytes Dendritic cells   Effector T cells

T lymphocytes

Complement NK cells

Hours	Days

0   6   12   1   4   7
Time after infection

infections. However, many pathogenic microbes have evolved to resist innate immunity, and their elimination requires the more powerful mechanisms of adaptive immunity. There are many connections between the innate and adaptive immune systems. The innate immune response to microbes stimulates adaptive immune responses and influences the nature of the adaptive responses. Conversely, adaptive immune responses often work by enhancing the protective mechanisms of innate immunity, making them capable of effectively combating pathogenic microbes.

Task 1 **Find out the answers to the following questions and then compare your answers with a partner.**

1. What kind of defense mechanisms does innate immunity consist of?

2. What are the defining characteristics of adaptive immunity?

3. Why is adaptive immune system called specific immunity?

4. What is the definition of antigen according to the passage?

5. Since there is innate immunity, why is adaptive immunity called for to defend against infection?

Task 2 You will hear 20 words or phrases which will be read three times. Write them down on the blanks and check with your partner after you finish.

1. _____   2. _____   3. _____   4. _____

5. _____   6. _____   7. _____   8. _____

9. _____   10. _____   11. _____   12. _____

13. _____   14. _____   15. _____   16. _____

17. _____   18. _____   19. _____   20. _____

Task 3 You are going to hear a passage which will be read three times. Take some notes while you are listening to the passage and then answer the following questions.

1. When does cytokine storm occur?

_____

2. What foods can be helpful in calming a cytokine storm?

_____

3. What needs to be noted before treating with cytokine blockers?

_____

Part III   Oral Presentation and Discussion

Task 4 Read the following passage and make an oral presentation.

Understanding How Vaccines Work

Vaccines help develop immunity by imitating an infection. This type of infection, however, does not cause illness, but it does cause the immune system to produce T-lymphocytes and antibodies. Sometimes, after getting a vaccine, the imitation infection can cause minor symptoms, such as fever. Such minor symptoms are normal and should be expected as the body builds immunity. Once the imitation infection goes away, the body is left with a supply of "memory" T-lymphocytes, as well as B-lymphocytes that will remember how to fight that disease in the future. However, it typically takes a few weeks for the body to produce T-lymphocytes and B-lymphocytes after vaccination. Therefore, it is possible that a person who was infected with a disease just before or just after vaccination could develop symptoms and get a disease, because the vaccine has not had enough time to provide protection.

Types of Vaccines

Scientists take many approaches to designing vaccines. These approaches are based on information about the germs (viruses or bacteria) the vaccine will prevent, such as how it infects cells and how the immune system responds to it. Practical considerations, such as regions of the world where the vaccine would be used, are also important because the strain of a virus and environmental conditions, such as temperature and risk of exposure, may be different in various parts of the world. The vaccine delivery options available may also differ geographically. Today there are five main types of vaccines that infants and young children commonly receive:

• Live, attenuated vaccines fight viruses. These vaccines contain a version of the living virus that has been weakened so that it does not cause serious disease in people with healthy immune systems. Because live, attenuated vaccines are the closest thing to a natural infection, they are good teachers for the immune system. Examples of live, attenuated vaccines include measles, mumps, and rubella vaccine (MMR) and varicella (chickenpox) vaccine. Even though these vaccines are very effective, not everyone can receive them. Children with weakened immune systems—for example, those who are undergoing chemotherapy—cannot get live vaccines.

• Inactivated vaccines also fight viruses. These vaccines are made by inactivating, or killing, the virus during the process of making the vaccine. The inactivated polio vaccine is an example of this type of vaccine. Inactivated vaccines produce immune responses in different ways than live, attenuated vaccines. Often, multiple doses are necessary to build up and/or maintain immunity.

• Toxoid vaccines prevent diseases caused by bacteria that produce toxins (poisons) in the body. In the process of making these vaccines, the toxins are weakened so they cannot cause illness. Weakened toxins are called toxoids. When the immune system receives a vaccine containing a toxoid, it learns how to fight off the natural toxin. The DTaP vaccine contains diphtheria and tetanus toxoids.

• Subunit vaccines include only parts of the virus or bacteria, or subunits, instead of the entire germ. Because these vaccines contain only the essential antigens and not all the other molecules that make up the germ, side effects are less common. The pertussis (whooping cough) component of the DTaP vaccine is an example of a subunit vaccine.

• Conjugate vaccines fight a different type of bacteria. These bacteria have antigens with an outer coating of sugar-like substances called polysaccharides. This type of coating disguises the antigen, making it hard for a young child's immature immune system to recognize it and respond to it. Conjugate vaccines are effective for these types of bacteria because they connect (or conjugate) the polysaccharides to antigens that the immune system responds to very well. This linkage helps the immature immune system react to the coating and develop an immune response. An example of this type of vaccine is the Haemophilus influenzae type B (Hib) vaccine.

Vaccines Require More Than One Dose

There are four reasons that babies—and even teens or adults for that matter—who receive a vaccine for the first time may need more than one dose:

• For some vaccines (primarily inactivated vaccines), the first dose does not provide as much immunity as possible. So, more than one dose is needed to build more complete immunity. The vaccine that protects against the bacteria Hib, which causes meningitis, is a good example.

• In other cases, such as the DTaP vaccine, which protects against diphtheria, tetanus, and pertussis, the initial series of four shots that children receive as part of their infant immunizations helps them build immunity. After a while, however, that immunity begins to wear off. At that point, a "booster" dose is needed to bring immunity levels back up. This booster dose is needed at 4 years through 6 years old for DTaP. Another booster against these diseases is needed at 11 years or 12 years of age. This booster for older children—and teens and adults, too—is called Tdap.

• For some vaccines (primarily live vaccines), studies have shown that more than one dose is needed for everyone to develop the best immune response. For example, after one dose of the MMR vaccine, some people may not develop enough antibodies to fight off infection. The second dose helps make sure that almost everyone is protected.

• Finally, in the case of the flu vaccine, adults and children (older than 6 months) need to get a dose every year. Children 6 months through 8 years old who have never gotten the flu vaccine in the past or have only gotten one dose in past years need two doses the first year they are vaccinated against flu for best protection. Then, annual flu shots are needed because the disease-causing viruses may be different from year to year. Every year, the flu vaccine is designed to prevent the specific viruses that experts predict will be circulating.

Task 5 Theme-related discussion.

Vaccines are vital in making progress against infectious diseases and saving millions of lives every year. However, there are still some worries about the safety and effectiveness of vaccines. For example, vaccines offer strong protection, but that protection takes time to build. People must take all the required doses of a vaccine to build complete immunity.

Please watch the MOOC, think about it, and discuss the following questions with your partner.

1. What are the primary challenges to vaccination?

2. How can the safety and effectiveness of vaccines be improved to protect vulnerable populations better?

Part Ⅳ Word Formation

immunity［英］免疫

  immun(o)-［希］免疫

    immunocompetence /ˌɪmjuːnəʊˈkɒmpɪtəns/ n . 免疫活性

    immunocyte /ˌɪmjuːnəʊˈsaɪt/ n . 免疫细胞

    immunodeficiency /ˌɪmjuːnəʊdɪˈfɪʃənsi/ n . 免疫缺损

over［英］高

  hyper-［希］过多,过度,超过

    hyperadrenalism /ˌhaɪpərəˈdriːnəlɪzəm/ n . 肾上腺功能亢进

    hyperglycemia /ˌhaɪpəglaɪˈsiːmiə/ n . 高血糖,血糖过多

    hyperlipidemia /ˈhaɪpəˌlɪpɪˈdiːmiə/ n . 高脂血症,血脂过多

lymph［英］淋巴

  lymph(o)-［希］淋巴

    lymphocyte /ˈlɪmfəʊsaɪt/ n . 淋巴细胞

    lymphangitis /ˌlɪmfænˈdʒaɪtɪs/ n . 淋巴管炎

    lymphology /lɪmˈfɒlədʒi/ n . 淋巴学

white［英］白

  leuk(o)-［希］白,白细胞

    leukemia /ljuːˈkiːmiə/ n . 白血病

    leukoderma /ˌljuːkəʊˈdɜːmə/ n . 白斑病

    leukoencephalitis /ˌljuːkəʊenˌsefəˈlaɪtɪs/ n . 白质脑炎

nerve［英］神经

  neur(o)-［希］神经

    neurobiology /ˌnjʊərəʊbaɪˈɒlədʒi/ n . 神经生物学

    neurocirculatory /ˌnjʊərəʊˈsɜːkjʊlətəri/ adj . 神经(与)循环系统的

    neurodermatitis /ˈnjʊərəʊˌdɜːməˈtaɪtɪs/ n . 神经性皮肤炎

hearing［英］听(觉)

  acou-［希］听(觉)的

    acousma /əˈkuːsmə/ n . 幻听,听幻觉

    acoustics /əˈkuːstɪks/ n . 声学

    acoustigram /əˈkuːstɪgræm/ n . 关节音像图

deficiency［英］不足,缺少

  -penia［希］减少,缺乏

erythropenia /ɪˌrɪθrəʊˈpiːnɪə/ *n*. 红细胞减少

glycopenia /ˌglaɪkəʊˈpiːnɪə/ *n*. 低血糖，血糖过少

leukopenia /ˌljuːkəˈpiːnɪə/ *n*. 白细胞减少

Task 6 **Match each of the following terms with its definition.**

1	lymph nodes	A	the graphic tracing of the curves of sounds produced by the motion of a joint
2	immunoglobulin	B	an abnormal increase in the number of white blood cells in the blood
3	acoustigram	C	a genetic disorder characterized by multiple tumors of the nerve trunks
4	hyperemia	D	bean-shaped masses of tissue where white blood cells are formed
5	leukocytosis	E	an excess of blood within an organ or tissue
6	neurofibromatosis	F	any of a set of serum glycoproteins which show antibody activity

Task 7 **Fill in the blanks with words or phrases given in the box. Change the form where necessary.**

hyperpnea	immune evasion	neuralgia	acoustic
immunological tolerance	glycopenia	leukemia	lymphocyte
neuron	leukocyte		

1. If you are frequently experiencing severe stabbing or burning pain, then you may have a damaged or irritated nerve. This type of pain is known as _____ , and it can occur throughout the body and face.

2. There are two main types of _____ : T cells, which control your body's immune system response, and B cells, which make antibodies.

3. Our ear drums register vibrations or _____ waves moving through the air as sound.

4. _____ is the process by which immune cells are made unresponsive to self-antigens to prevent damage to healthy tissues.

5. _____ is a cancer of the blood, characterized by the rapid growth of abnormal blood cells. This uncontrolled growth takes place in your bone marrow.

6. _____ carry signals throughout the central and peripheral nervous systems.

7. White blood cells, also known as _____ , are responsible for protecting your

body from infection.

8. Pathogenic organisms and tumors use the strategy of _____ to evade a host's immune response.

9. Blood glucose or tissue glucose below 3.9 mmol/L is regarded as hypoglycemia or _____ .

10. Possible causes of _____ , which involves taking deeper or larger breaths than usual, range from high altitude to heart failure.

Part Ⅴ   Fast Reading

Vertebrate Immune System

The survival of members of most vertebrate species to an age at which they can reproduce depends critically on their ability to resist infection. The specialized cells and organs that protect these animals from infection and death make up the immune system. This system continuously monitors every tissue and organ in the body for invaders. When the presence of cells or molecules that "do not belong" is confirmed, the immune system activates a battery of weapons designed to eliminate or contain the source of the infection. Growing awareness about inherited and acquired immunodeficiency diseases has helped underscore how absolutely crucial this protective system is for our survival.

The study of immunology, as distinguished from other areas of biology, revolves around two central questions. How does the immune system recognize the enormous variety of foreign shapes that must be targeted in order to ensure survival? How do we manage to discriminate between self structures and shapes that are foreign? The explosion in our knowledge of immunology at the molecular and cellular level has considerably simplified our understanding of the immune system. As a result, it is now possible to describe immunological phenomena such as the "generation of diversity" and "self-nonself recognition" in fairly simple cellular and molecular terms.

The primary goal of the immune system is to protect us from disease. One cannot seriously discuss this subject without reference to disorders that result either from the absence of an immune response or from an immune response gone away. In this course we will briefly look at a number of diseases largely from a mechanistic point of view. Indeed there is little doubt that we are likely to witness a new era in which an increased understanding of immune function will contribute to novel therapeutic approaches to immunodeficiency diseases, organ transplantation and cancer. Understanding the immune system may open the door to a very exciting and intriguing world.

Innate Immunity

The immune system as we know it in its highly evolved form is extraordinarily versatile. A considerably simpler version existed before the evolution of vertebrates. This more ancient immune system represents the principal defense machinery in invertebrates (animals such as insects and worms, which lack a backbone). The basic elements of this early protective system have been preserved in all animals including man. This primitive system, now frequently described as the "innate" immune system, is made up primarily of proteins called agglutinins and cells called phagocytes.

One of the underlying principles in nature's grand design for host defense is the requirement that the immune system should discriminate between self and "non-self".

Agglutinins are multivalent proteins which recognize structures that are not found on host cells but which are commonly found on the surface of microorganisms. The term multivalent here refers to the presence of more than one recognition site in a single protein. Having more than one recognition site allows agglutinins to "agglutinate" or clump target cells such as bacteria with the appropriate coat sugar for instance. An agglutinin which recognizes carbohydrates is called a lectin. Lectins that are capable of specifically agglutinating certain microbes are secreted by cells of the host. These lectins do not recognize sugars on the surface of host cells and thereby discriminate between self and non-self. Phagocytes (phagos = to eat) are specialized cells which engulf invading microorganisms. They either use specific receptors which discriminate between self and foreign shapes or they recognize microbes that have been coated by host agglutinins.

Another important component of the innate immune system is a set of circulating complement proteins. These proteins obtain their name from their ability to complement the function of antibody molecules in the immune system. They help destroy target cells coated by antibody proteins by punching holes in the cell membrane. The concentration of sodium chloride outside cells is relatively high—the holes in the membrane permit salt and water to rush into targets cells which swell up and burst, a process known as lysis. Complement proteins however existed in invertebrates before the evolution of antibodies. A subset of complement proteins can directly coat certain bacteria, thus either lysing them or targeting them for ingestion by phagocytes. The complement system will be discussed in a subsequent lecture.

Vertebrate Immune Systems Recognize a Tremendous Diversity of Shapes

The innate immune system has remained valuable over millions of years of evolution. We, as a species, retain this machinery as a first line of defense even though we possess a superimposed and more refined system for host protection. This more sophisticated and specific immune system evolved in vertebrates probably because the innate immune system could not effectively guarantee the survival of creatures with a longer potential life span.

The earliest vertebrates were very primitive fish and it is in these animals that the evolution of the immune system made a quantum leap. The immune system in its highly evolved form permits the specific recognition of an incredible variety of shapes that are identified as being foreign. Acquired or specific immunity as seen in vertebrates, is designed to be able to deal with any conceivable foreign shape that nature can present or that any synthetic chemist may choose to create at any time in the future. A particularly interesting characteristic of vertebrate immune systems is their ability to respond more readily to foreign shapes that they have seen before, a phenomenon known as immunological memory.

Lymphocytes and the Clonal Selection Hypothesis

A major strategy in the evolution of vertebrate immune systems was the development of a means to synthesize a tremendous repertoire of distinct molecules that can recognize and thus help dispose of an almost infinite variety of pathogens. The cells responsible for the vast repertoire of the immune system, so far referred to as immune cells, are known as lymphocytes. One lineage of lymphocytes develops in the bone marrow of most vertebrates and in a specialized organ in birds known as the bursa of Fabricius. These lymphocytes are known as B lymphocytes (for bursal or bone-marrow derived).

Each individual B lymphocyte makes a distinct protein known as an antibody molecule which can recognize a different shape from those recognized by other antibodies made by other B cells. An antigen is most simply defined as any structure that can be recognized by the immune system. A given antigen may trigger the expansion of a specific B cell expressing the appropriate antibody molecule on the cell surface. This type of distinct antibody molecule expressed on the cell surface is known as an antigen receptor or a membrane immunoglobulin.

Each antigen receptor bearing cell may expand on exposure to a cognate antigen to form a clone of B lymphocytes that secrete a specific antibody molecule. The concept of distinct antibodies being synthesized by individual lymphocytes which can be clonally expanded by a specific cognate antigen was proposed by Burnet and Talmage in 1955. The clonal selection theory is a central paradigm of vertebrate immunology.

While it is useful to think of the immune system as an army of lymphocytes primed to recognize and destroy invaders, we now appreciate that this is not a faceless army, but a force made up of highly specialized individual soldiers. When an invader enters the body, the majority of lymphocytes it encounters may be totally impervious to its existence. The few specialized lymphocytes with the "right" receptors that specifically recognize antigenic shapes on the invader are stimulated. They respond by proliferating (clonal expansion) and also activate an impressive battery of weapons designed to wipe out this pathogen.

Task 8 Read the passage and decide whether the statements are true or false. If it is true, write "T". If it is not, write "F".

1. Inherited and acquired immunodeficiency diseases are absolutely crucial for our survival. ( )

2. Innate immune system is preserved in animals except man. ( )

3. Vertebrate immune systems can guarantee the survival of creatures with a longer potential life span. ( )

4. Immune system can be considered as an army of lymphocytes primed to recognize and destroy invaders. ( )

5. The primary goal of the immune system is to open the door to a very exciting and intriguing world. ( )

Task 9 Please read the passage again and write a two-hundred-word synopsis.

Part Ⅵ   Translation

Task 10 Analyze the following sentences and then put them into Chinese.

1. The defining characteristics of adaptive immunity are exquisite specificity for distinct molecules and an ability to "remember" and respond more vigorously to repeated exposures to the same microbe.

_____

2. Therefore, it is possible that a person who was infected with a disease just before or just after vaccination could develop symptoms and get a disease, because the vaccine has not had enough time to provide protection.

_____

3. While it is useful to think of the immune system as an army of lymphocytes primed to recognize and destroy invaders, we now appreciate that this is not a faceless army, but a force made up of highly specialized individual soldiers.

_____

平行结构

两个或者两个以上意思并列的句子成分应该采用同等的语法结构,即平行结构,这可以使表达更清晰流畅、简明易懂。但是,英文翻译与写作中经常会出现以下错误结构:

例 1 Many people choose the first therapy because it is fast, offers convenience, and it is not very expensive.

本句中 because 后面列举的都是原因,意思是并列的,使用的语法结构却各不相同,有形容词、动宾结构,还有完整的句子,应修改为同等的语法结构,如全部使用形容词形式,可修改如下:

Many people choose the first therapy because it is <u>fast, convenient and inexpensive.</u>

例 2 He invested his money in stocks, in real estate, and a home for retired performers.

可修改为:

He invested his money <u>in stocks, in real estate, and in a home for retired performers.</u>(都用"in + 名词"结构)

判断平行结构是否使用正确,可通过补加共有成分来检查各个并列成分是否保持一致。例 2 中,invested his money 是共有成分,补加后此例语法结构仍然正确:He invested his money in stocks,(invested his money)in real estate, and(invested his money)in a home for retired performers.

国内医学生在进行医学英语摘要的写作与翻译时,常常忽视平行结构的使用。

例 3 Aim: <u>To investigate</u> the molecular mechanism of berberine in ameliorating insulin resistance and treating type 2 diabetes mellitus(T2DM), the effect of berberine on PI-3K and GLUT4 protein expression in skeletal muscle of T2DM rat models <u>were observed.</u>

上例作者的本意是用动词不定式来表达研究目的,但却使用了不定式和主谓式两种不同的语法形式,造成结构上的不平行,不符合英语的表达习惯,应修改为:

Aim: <u>To investigate</u> the molecular mechanism of berberine in ameliorating insulin resistance and treating type 2 diabetes mellitus(T2DM), and <u>to observe</u> the effect of berberine on PI-3K and GLUT4 protein expression in skeletal muscle of T2DM rat models.

英语语句常借助 and、but、or 等并列连词连接同等的语法结构,可通过定位分析这些词语的上下文结构来判断是否使用了正确的平行结构。此外,在英文摘要中使用平行结构还要注意以下几点：

（1）不含并列意思的句子成分不能采用平行结构。

误　PTP1B was <u>subcloned</u> with primers containing restriction endonucleases recognition sites of BamH I and EcoR I，ligated into pET-28a（＋），<u>transduced into</u> DE3，induced with IPTG，and <u>analyzed with</u> SDS-PAGE and Western blot.

正　PTP1B <u>was subcloned</u> with primers containing restriction endonucleases recognition sites of BamH I and EcoR I，ligated into pET-28a（＋），transduced into DE3，induced with IPTG and <u>expressed proteins were analyzed with</u> SDS-PAGE and Western blot.

克隆载体 PTP1B 测序后设计带酶切位点 BamH I 和 EcoR I 的引物，PCR 后酶切连入 pET-28a（＋）中，转化 DE3，IPTG 诱导表达，SDS-PAGE 后用蛋白印迹法检测其特异表达。

（2）平行结构中同等的语法结构包括名词、不定式、动名词、介词短语和从句等，它们在平行结构中的使用应保持一致，不可混用。平行结构中的各个成分保持一致，还包括介词（in、on、by、with）、冠词（the、a、an）、助动词（had、has、would）和人称代词（his、her、our）等的一致。

例：心电图限于 T 波改变，表现为：（1）振幅增加，波顶尖或基底增宽；（2）双峰；（3）平坦或倒置。

误：Electrocardiographic changes were limited to the T wave：（1）<u>increase</u>（名词）in amplitude，assuming a "spinous" appearance，or broad at the base，（2）<u>double peaked or "cloven"</u>（形容词），and（3）flat or inverted T <u>waves</u>（名词）.

正：Electrocardiographic changes were limited to the T wave，which may be：（1）<u>increased</u>（形容词）in amplitude，assuming a "spinous" appearance，or broad at the base，（2）<u>double-peaked or "cloven"</u>（形容词），and（3）<u>flat or inverted</u>（形容词）.

Task 11 Translate the following sentences into English.

1. 最常出现的症状是咳嗽、胸痛、哮鸣（wheeze）、体重减轻、咯血（hemoptysis）及气短。

2. 搭桥术（bypass）的结果显示仅 24％效果良好，42％满意，34％不满意。

3. 几乎所有的脓胸患者（empyemas）都需要切除小段肋骨（a rib resection）或去骨膜（decortication）进行外科引流手术。

4. 所随访的患者无死亡，无严重并发症，无垂体功能低下（hypopituitarism）。

5. 检查肝功能指标，观察肝组织形态及肝细胞超微结构（ultrastructure）变化。

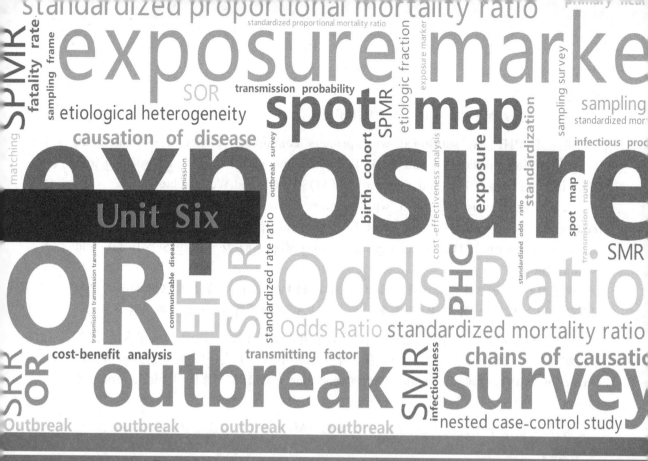

Unit Six

Epidemiology

✓课文音频
✓听力音频
✓在线课程
✓课件申请

Epidemiology and Its Applications

The word epidemiology comes from the Greek words *epi*, meaning on or upon, *demos*, meaning people, and *logos*, meaning the study of. In other words, the word epidemiology has its roots in the study of what befalls a population. Epidemiology is a scientific discipline with sound methods of scientific inquiry at its foundation. It is data-driven and relies on a systematic and unbiased approach to the collection, analysis, and interpretation of data. Basic epidemiologic methods tend to rely on careful observation and use of valid comparison groups to assess whether what was observed, such as the number of cases of disease in a particular area during a particular time period or the frequency of an exposure among persons with disease, differs from what might be expected.

epidemiology /ˌepɪˌdiːmiˈɒlədʒi/ *n.* 传染病学,流行病学

Epidemiologists assume that illness does not occur randomly in a population, but happens only when the right accumulation of risk factors or determinants exists in an individual. To search for these determinants, epidemiologists use analytic epidemiology or epidemiologic studies to provide the "Why" and "How" of such events. They assess whether groups with different rates of disease differ in their demographic characteristics, genetic or immunologic make-up, behaviors, environmental exposures, or other so-called potential risk factors. Ideally, the findings provide sufficient evidence to direct prompt and effective public health control and prevention measures.

randomly /ˈrændəmli/ *adv.* 任意地,随机地
determinant /dɪˈtɜːmɪnənt/ *n.* 决定因素

demographic /ˌdiːməˈɡræfɪk/ *adj.* 人口统计学的

Epidemiology and the information generated by epidemiologic methods have been used in many ways. Some common uses are described below.

Assessing the Community's Health

Public health officials responsible for policy development, implementation, and evaluation use epidemiologic information as a factual framework for decision making. To assess the health of a population or community, relevant sources of data must be identified and analyzed by person, place, and time. Sometimes, more detailed data may need to be collected and analyzed to determine whether health services are available, accessible, effective, and efficient.

Making Individual Decisions

Many individuals may not realize that they use epidemiologic information to make daily decisions affecting their health. When persons decide to quit smoking, climb the stairs rather than wait for an elevator, eat a salad rather than a cheeseburger with fries for lunch, or use a **condom**, they may be influenced, consciously or unconsciously, by epidemiologists' assessment of risk. Many epidemiologic findings are directly relevant to the choices people make every day, choices that affect their health over a lifetime.

Completing the Clinical Picture

When investigating a disease outbreak, epidemiologists rely on health-care providers and laboratorians to establish the proper diagnosis of individual patients. But epidemiologists also contribute to physicians' understanding of the clinical picture and natural history of disease. For example, in late 1989, a physician saw three patients with unexplained **eosinophilia**(an increase in the number of a specific type of white blood cell called an eosinophilia) and **myalgia** (severe muscle pains). Although the physician could not make a definitive diagnosis, he notified public health authorities. Within weeks, epidemiologists had identified enough other cases to characterize the **spectrum** and course of the illness that came to be known as

condom /'kɒndəm/ n. 避孕套,安全套

eosinophilia /iːəˌsɪnəˈfɪliə/ n. 嗜曙红细胞过多,嗜曙红细胞增多
myalgia /maɪˈældʒiə/ n. 肌痛

spectrum /'spektrəm/ n. 系列,范围;光谱

eosinophilia-myalgia syndrome.

Searching for Causes

Much epidemiologic research is devoted to searching for causal factors that influence one's risk of disease. Ideally, the goal is to identify a cause so that appropriate public health action might be taken. One can argue that epidemiology can never prove a causal relationship between an exposure and a disease, since much of epidemiology is based on ecologic reasoning. Nevertheless, epidemiology often provides enough information to support effective action. Examples date from the removal of the handle from the Broad St. Pump following John Snow's investigation of cholera in the Golden Square area of London in 1854, to the withdrawal of a vaccine against rotavirus in 1999 after epidemiologists found that it increased the risk of intussusception, a potentially life-threatening condition. Just as often, epidemiology and laboratory science converge to provide the evidence needed to establish causation.

cholera /ˈkɒlərə/ n. 霍乱

vaccine /ˈvæksiːn/ n. 疫苗

intussusception /ˌɪntəsəˈsepʃən/ n. 肠套叠

causation /kɔːˈzeɪʃən/ n. 因果关系

Task 1 Find out the answers to the following questions and then compare your answers with a partner.

1. How is the term "epidemiology" defined?

2. What are the basic epidemiologic methods mentioned in the passage?

3. What is the significance of the findings of epidemiologic study?

4. According to the passage, are many epidemiologic findings directly relevant to the choices people make every day?

5. What do epidemiologists usually do when investigating a disease outbreak?

Part Ⅱ   Listening

Task 2 You will hear 20 words or phrases which will be read three times. Write them down on the blanks and check with your partner after you finish.

1. _____   2. _____   3. _____   4. _____

5. _____   6. _____   7. _____   8. _____

9. _____   10. _____   11. _____   12. _____

13. _____   14. _____   15. _____   16. _____

17. _____   18. _____   19. _____   20. _____

Task 3 You are going to hear a passage which will be read three times. Take some notes while you are listening to the passage and then answer the following questions.

1. What are the findings of an epidemiological survey used for?

_____

2. Who will be interviewed in an epidemiological survey?

_____

3. What may be recorded on a survey map?

_____

Part Ⅲ   Oral Presentation and Discussion

Task 4 Read the following passage and make an oral presentation.

Modernizing Epidemic Science: Enabling Patient-Centered Research During Epidemics

Background

Emerging and epidemic infectious diseases (EEIDs) have shaped society, and recent events affirm that they will continue to do so. In less than two years, Ebola virus disease (EVD) and the Zika virus prompted the World Health Organization (WHO) to declare Public Health Emergencies of International Concern. Meanwhile, the Middle East respiratory syndrome coronavirus (MERS-CoV) continues to cause sporadic cases and nosocomial outbreaks, and an increasing diversity of avian influenza viruses are infecting people across numerous continents.

Preparing ourselves adequately for these threats demands action on many fronts. Patient-centered research needs to be included as one key pillar of an enhanced outbreak investigation, response, and control system. Patients are the primary source of much of the information (e. g. clinical presentation and outcomes) and materials (e. g. pathogens and antibodies) that are vital for both clinical and public health decision-making, for advancing basic scientific understanding, and for evaluating the products of enhanced diagnostic, drug and vaccine development pipelines.

The Importance of Patient-Centred Research During Epidemics

1) Improving patient outcomes

In the turmoil of epidemics and the pressure to protect public health and economic interests, it is sometimes forgotten that patients lie at the heart of every outbreak. These patients, their families, and the clinical teams caring for them often struggle with frightening uncertainty and inadequate support and resources. However, during epidemics, decisions such as which drugs, fluids, or supportive care strategies to offer patients are usually made ad hoc by the treating clinician or from guidelines that approximate other diseases and experiences. The African trial of Fluid Expansion As Supportive Therapy (FEAST) for critically ill children, which found that giving fluid boluses to severely ill children with impaired perfusion in resource-limited settings in Africa actually increased mortality, was a clear demonstration of the potential dangers of plausible extrapolation.

2) Helping to control the epidemic

Patients with epidemic and emerging infections deserve to benefit from the fruits of research as much as any other patient. However, the broader societal benefits of clinical research are even greater in the context of outbreaks. A well-focused and calibrated public health response to an epidemic can save lives and money. Many aspects of an appropriate public health response depend on high-quality data and samples from patients. For example, reliable illness severity data are required to predict the number of infected and ill people and then scale the response appropriately; groups at high risk for infection or poor prognosis need to be identified for targeted preventative and treatment interventions; genetic sequencing of pathogens from biological samples can provide critical information on transmission pathways, evolutionary pressures, and drug resistance.

How Do We Make Progress?

1) Integrated clinical data capture

Currently, outbreak response characterized by an artificial separation of the public health, clinical, and scientific response is an understandable consequence of engrained disciplinary divisions and regulatory frameworks. However, it could be more inefficient given that the ultimate aims of all groups are to improve patient outcomes and control the epidemic. Under even a cursory examination, it is clear that the boundaries between the public health, clinical, and scientific response are blurred, with the necessary evidence overlapping and being collected from the same patient. What distinguishes research from clinical or public health practice is often difficult to define, and rather than trying to draw arbitrary boundaries, we should aim to integrate the data needs of all disciplines. The quality of evidence could be improved by designing unified data and sample collection protocols driven by an explicit link to the public health and clinical decisions that need to be taken.

2) New clinical study methodologies and tools

Significant improvements in the care provided for patients treated for battlefield trauma and in pre-hospital settings over the last few decades demonstrate that it is feasible to conduct patient-centered research in austere and challenging environments. The biggest remaining challenge for clinical research on EEIDs is uncertainty: emerging infections are often relatively rare; understanding of the clinical presentation and natural history is usually limited; and outbreaks are unpredictable in timing, location, and size. Classical clinical trial designs that require predictable and often large case numbers to test hypotheses need to be better suited to this epidemiological uncertainty. Trial designs are needed that are robust to uncertainties in the number, timing, and location of cases; clinical phenotype, progression, and outcomes; the optimal comparison (control) group; and the optimal intervention to test.

3) Strengthened global coordination and support for clinical research on EEIDs

It is worth considering the substantial difficulties that face those who wish to undertake clinical research on emerging and epidemic infections. First, many emerging pathogens might be considered rare. The diseases currently under the "rare diseases" umbrella are largely severe non-communicable diseases with a genetic component. Second, the timeframe for action can be both unpredictable and extremely short, with the average duration of influenza epidemics being ten weeks, with the peak incidence reached after only four weeks. Third, the spatial distribution can be widespread. The bottom line is that the unpredictability, rapidity, and rarity of many emerging infectious disease outbreaks render it improbable that a meaningful research response can be delivered by isolated investigators or institutions. Large-scale international collaboration is essential.

Conclusion

The response to epidemics has been plagued with poor data and weak evidence, and the central importance of patient-based clinical research is widely underappreciated. We risk continuing to fail the patients and communities most affected unless we work towards an improved framework. Key features of this improved framework include integrating patient-centered research with other aspects of outbreak response, developing methods and tools that address the genuine epidemiological and contextual challenges of EEIDs, and building an organizational model for clinical research on EEIDs that is effective and sustainable.

Task 5 **Theme-related discussion.**

An epidemic is a major incident that occurs suddenly and causes or may cause severe damage to public health, which is emergent in time and lasting in influence. There have been many pandemics in human history, like the Black Death, the 1918 Influenza Pandemic, and the AIDS pandemic, which caused intense public panic.

Please watch the MOOC, think about it, and discuss the following questions with your partner.

1. What are the scientific measures to prevent respiratory infectious diseases?

2. In the face of the Plague and the Black Death, how did medical professionals believe in science and abolish superstitions?

Part Ⅳ Word Formation

cholera [英] 霍乱

　cholera- [希] 霍乱
　　choleragen /ˈkɒlərədʒən/ n. 霍乱原
　　choleraic /kɒləˈreɪɪk/ adj. 霍乱的
　　choleraphage /ˈkɒlərəfeɪdʒ/ n. 霍乱噬菌体

eosin [英] 伊红，曙红

　eosin- [希] 伊红，曙红
　　eosinocyte /ˌiːəˈsɪnəsaɪt/ n. 伊红细胞，嗜酸细胞
　　eosinopenia /ˌiːəsɪnəˈpiːniə/ n. 伊红细胞减少，嗜酸细胞减少
　　eosinophil /ˌiːəˈsɪnəfɪl/ n. 伊红细胞，嗜酸性细胞

graph [英] 图，图表

　-graphy [希] 描记法
　　nephrography /nəˈfrɒgrəfi/ n. 肾 X 线造影术
　　cystography /sɪsˈtɒgrəfi/ n. 膀胱造影术

pneumocystography /ˌnjuːməʊsɪs'tɒgrəfi/ n. 膀胱充气造影术

pain [英] 痛

  -algia [希] 痛

    neuralgia /njʊə'ræld3iə/ n. 神经痛

    odontalgia /ˌɒdɒn'tæld3iə/ n. 牙痛

    rectalgia /rek'tæld3iə/ n. 直肠痛

small [英] 小

  micro- [希] 微小的

    microbe /'maɪkrəʊb/ n. 微生物，病菌

    microorganism /ˌmaɪkrəʊ'ɔːgənɪz(ə)m/ n. 微生物

    microscope /'maɪkrəʊskəʊp/ n. 显微镜

marrow [英] 骨髓

  myel(o)- [希] 骨髓，脊髓

    myeloid /'maɪəlɔɪd/ adj. 骨髓的；骨髓样的

    myelogenous /ˌmaɪə'lɒd3ənəs/ adj. 骨髓内形成的

    myelitis /ˌmaɪə'laɪtɪs/ n. 脊髓炎

ear [英] 耳

  auricul(o)- [拉] 耳；心房

    auriculotherapy /ɔːˌrɪkjuːləʊ'θerəpi/ n. 耳针疗法

    auricular /ɔː'rɪkjuːlə/ adj. 耳郭的，耳的

    auriculare /ɔːˌrɪkjʊ'lɛə/ n. 耳道点

Task 6 **Match each of the following terms with its definition.**

1	nephralgia	A	the cholera enterotoxin
2	eosinophil	B	a malignant tumor formed by the cells of the bone marrow
3	myeloma	C	a leucocyte with a multilobed nucleus and coarse granular cytoplasm
4	choleragen	D	investigation of minute objects using a microscope
5	microscopy	E	pain in a kidney
6	pneumocystography	F	radiography of the bladder following injection of air

Task 7 **Fill in the blanks with words or phrases given in the box. Change the form where necessary.**

epidemic	cholera	cystography	gastralgia
microbe	odontalgia	auriculoventricular	microscopic
auriculotherapy	myelitis		

1. If tooth decay is the cause of your _____, a filling may be used to fill in the decayed area and prevent further damage.

2. The _____ valves are located between the atria and the ventricles of the heart.

3. _____ is an acute diarrheal illness caused by infection of the intestine with Vibrio cholerae bacteria.

4. The patient described the _____ as a sharp, burning sensation that worsened after eating spicy foods.

5. Other forms of _____ other than ear seeds include ear acupuncture, in which tiny needles are placed in the ears.

6. _____ is a diagnostic procedure or an imaging test done to diagnose the problems of the urinary bladder.

7. The _____ examination of the blood sample revealed abnormal cell growth.

8. Transverse _____ is a neurological condition that happens when both sides of the same section of the spinal cord become inflamed.

9. The rise and decline in _____ prevalence of an infectious disease is a probability phenomenon dependent upon the transfer of an effective dose of the infectious agent from an infected individual to a susceptible one.

10. Microorganisms or _____ are microscopic creatures that are invisible to the naked eye.

Part V　Fast Reading

Monkeypox

Introduction

Monkeypox virus was first isolated in late 1958 in Copenhagen during two outbreaks of a small pox-like disease in a colony of cynomolgus monkeys. No clinical signs were noted before the eruptive phase of the disease, which was characterized by a maculopapular rash. The virus was named monkeypox virus because of its close similarity to other known poxviruses.

Between 1960 and 1968, several other outbreaks of monkeypox were reported in colonies of captive monkeys in the United States and the Netherlands. No cases were detected in humans during these outbreaks, despite the deaths of many affected animals, which suggested that humans were not susceptible to monkeypox. The first case of monkeypox in humans was reported in 1970 as part of the national smallpox surveillance and eradication program in Africa. Between September 1970 and March 1971, six additional cases of monkeypox were identified in humans in West African countries. Most of these patients were young children, and none had been vaccinated against smallpox.

Monkeypox in humans remained an exclusively African disease, with sporadic cases diagnosed in forested areas of Central or West Africa and small outbreaks mainly in the Democratic Republic of Congo until 2003 when the first cases outside Africa were reported. These cases occurred in the United States and were linked to the importation of Gambian pouched rats from Ghana to Texas. The rodents transmitted the virus to prairie dogs housed in the same exotic-animal facility, and the prairie dogs then infected humans, mostly young adults and children. In 2018, five infected patients were identified: three in the United Kingdom, one in Israel, and one in Singapore. These imported cases were linked to persons from Nigeria, where a large outbreak occurred in 2017—2018. The disease has continued to be common in Africa, with rare sporadic cases in the United Kingdom and the United States.

In May 2022, a series of monkeypox cases was identified in the United Kingdom, Portugal, and Italy, mostly involving men who have sex with men. Health authorities rapidly established that this series was the start of a new outbreak. Given the unusual geographic distribution of cases, the World Health Organization (WHO) and other public health institutions raised the alert as early as May 16, 2022. The current outbreak is due to what we have termed clade three monkeypox viruses (derived from the West African clade). The WHO declared a global health emergency on July 23, 2022.

Clinical Features

It is probably too early to provide a precise description of the clinical aspects of this monkeypox outbreak. However, they seem to mostly match the clinical features of classic outbreaks described above, with some differences, a combination that has led to a new pattern—a U. K. Health Security Agency analysis of national cases in this outbreak estimated the mean incubation period at 9.22 days. A WHO analysis of data from 660 patients with at least one type of classic prodromal symptoms showed that 71.4% of the patients presented with systemic symptoms (e. g., fever and headache), and 49.0% had a localized lymphadenopathy. In the same analysis, 97.7% of the patients had a rash during the eruptive phase, 70.5% had anogenital skin and mucosal lesions, and 7.0% had oral skin and mucosal lesions. In the current outbreak, however, lesions are also being observed without a prodromal phase in a large proportion of patients. In one analysis, 13.7% of patients presented with mucocutaneous manifestations in the absence of systemic features.

The number of skin lesions is highly variable, with some patients presenting with only a few painless lesions. The skin lesions also appear to be asynchronous, ranging from single or clustered spots to umbilicated papules with progressive central ulceration and, finally, scabs, in contrast to the previously described pattern of simultaneous progression. In addition, the pattern of skin lesions is unusual, often in genital, anal, and perianal areas, without the typical centrifugal distribution, and cases of proctitis and pharyngitis have also been described.

Previous studies have shown that the clade two monkeypox virus causes mild disease, with a case fatality ratio of less than 1%, which is consistent with the low rates of hospitalization and death reported in this outbreak. The hospitalization rate is estimated to be 5 to 10%. Hospitalizations are related to cellulitis, in particular involving the genital and perineal region; severe anal and digestive involvement with rectal pain, penile edema, severe angina, and epiglottitis; and ocular involvement with blepharitis, conjunctivitis, and keratitis. Two fatal cases that were recently reported in young, healthy, nonimmunocompromised MSM (men who have sex with men) appeared to be related to encephalitis; these cases are still under investigation.

Vaccination and Treatment

The treatments currently authorized for monkeypox are

tecovirimat in the United States and Europe and brincidofovir in the United States alone. Tecovirimat inhibits the orthopoxvirus protein, blocking cell-to-cell viral transmission. Although tecovirimat is approved for the treatment of smallpox in the United States, its use for monkeypox is based on an investigational new drug application, and the agent has not received full regulatory approval. The efficacy of tecovirimat has been shown in preclinical studies, including four pivotal studies in nonhuman primates showing that the drug provided 95% protection from death, as compared with placebo. Phase 1 and 2 clinical trials have assessed the safety and side-effect profile of tecovirimat in humans. A recent observational study involving a very small number of patients with monkeypox suggested that tecovirimat may reduce the duration of viral shedding and illness.

Brincidofovir inhibits the viral DNA polymerase. The efficacy of this agent in improving survival after infection has been shown in mice and rabbits. Its safety in humans was assessed in clinical trials for cytomegalovirus disease in recipients of hematopoietic stem-cell transplants. Brincidofovir has gastrointestinal and hepatic toxic effects, and its safety profile is inferior to that of tecovirimat.

Randomized clinical trials are needed to evaluate the efficacy of these drugs, regardless of their authorization status. The WHO and several countries are implementing such trials, especially with tecovirimat. This evaluation should be performed not only in the countries affected by the current outbreak but also in areas where the disease is endemic.

Summary

The gradual decline in immunity to smallpox may partly explain an increase in the incidence of monkeypox in some regions where the disease is endemic. However, the current epidemic reminds us that viral emergence is a permanent phenomenon without boundaries and is often unpredictable in its nature, target, and magnitude. This outbreak illustrates how a disease affecting one region of the world can have a strong effect on areas where it is not endemic, with different target populations and new clinical presentations. To thwart the continuation of the current monkeypox epidemic, both in the African areas where it is endemic and in newly affected regions, the priorities are clear: first, increase awareness and education of populations, especially at-risk groups, to prevent infection and reduce transmission and spread; second, develop rapid, sensitive point-of-care detection tests to improve diagnosis and, consequently, prevention; and third, evaluate the effectiveness of existing treatments, vaccines, and vaccination strategies and improve efforts to make vaccination and treatment available to all affected groups and regions.

Task 8 Read the passage and decide whether the statements are true or false. If it is true, write "T". If it is not, write "F".

1. The first case of monkeypox in humans was reported in 1971 in a child without being vaccinated against smallpox. ( )

2. Monkeypox in humans remained an exclusively African disease until 2003 when the first cases outside Africa were reported. ( )

3. In the current multicountry outbreak, however, lesions are also being observed without a prodromal phase in a large proportion of patients. ( )

4. Tecovirimat has gastrointestinal and hepatic toxic effects, and its safety profile is inferior to that of Brincidofovir in the treatment for monkeypox. ( )

5. Evaluating the effectiveness of existing treatments, vaccines, and vaccination strategies is a top priority in preventing monkeypox epidemic. ( )

Task 9 Read the passage again and write a two-hundred-word synopsis.

Part VI Translation

Task 10 Analyze the following sentences and then put them into Chinese.

1. Basic epidemiologic methods tend to rely on careful observation and use of valid comparison groups to assess whether what was observed, such as the number of cases of disease in a particular area during a particular time period or the frequency of an exposure among persons with disease, differs from what might be expected.

2. Examples date from the removal of the handle from the Broad St. Pump following John Snow's investigation of cholera in the Golden Square area of London in 1854, to the withdrawal of a vaccine against rotavirus in 1999 after epidemiologists found that it increased the risk of intussusception, a potentially life-threatening condition.

_____

_____

3. Key features of this improved framework include integrating patient-centered research with other aspects of outbreak response, developing methods and tools that address the genuine epidemiological and contextual challenges of EEIDs, and building an organizational model for clinical research on EEIDs that is effective and sustainable.

_____

_____

医学翻译技巧

强调—后移

英语在其发展过程中形成了相对固定的词序,其主要的五种基本句型充分反映了这种固定词序的特征。而有时因为表达的需要,可以变动固定词序,将某些成分后移,形成句尾重心,以达到强调的目的。本处讨论的后移,主要针对医学英语文体。由于被动结构的多处使用,充当名词词组的中心词后有时带有结构复杂或较长的后置定语或同位语,这时常将该定语或同位语移至句尾,与中心词分隔以保持句子结构的平衡。这种后置定语大多是介词短语、分词短语或定语从句。

1. 介词短语做后置定语

例 1 作者对有关年龄、性别、职业、家族史、饮食习惯、抽烟史、接触史一一作了登记。

译文 1 Data on age, gender, occupation, family history, diet habit, smoking and exposure history were recorded.

本句主语 data 后面紧跟的介词短语 on ...,是一个较长的后置定语,而谓语是一个很短的被动语态 were recorded。上述译文显得头重脚轻,所以,可以将这个介词短语充当的后置定语移至谓语后面,达到句子平衡的效果。

译文 2 Data were recorded on age, gender, occupation, family history, diet habit, smoking and exposure history.

2. 分词短语做后置定语

例 2 近 2 年,出版了很多报道这个实验结果的文献。

译文 1 Over the past 2 years, papers reporting the results of the experiment were published.

本句主语 papers 后面紧跟着的分词短语 reporting ... ，是一个较长的后置定语，而谓语是一个很短的被动语态 were published。上述译文显得头重脚轻，所以，可以将这个分词短语充当的后置定语移至谓语后面，达到句子平衡的效果。

译文 2　Over the past 2 years, papers were published <u>reporting the results of the experiment</u>.

3. 从句做后置定语

例 3　我们将报导冠状动脉及周围血管低血镁引起缺血性心脏猝死的资料。

译文 1　Data <u>which suggests that sudden death ischemic heart may be due to hypomagnesemia in and around the coronary arterial and arteriolar vessels</u> will be presented.

本句后置定语是一个较长的从句，谓语很短，可以将从句调至句尾。

译文 2　Data will be presented <u>which suggests that sudden death ischemic heart may be due to hypomagnesemia in and around the coronary arterial and arteriolar vessels</u>.

4. 同位语从句后移

例 4　有证据表明，植物纤维对人类的营养吸收颇有影响，因为它们能使很多营养物质的吸收与代谢发生变化。

译文 1　Evidence <u>that plant fibers have profound influences on human nutrition because they alter the absorption and metabolism of many nutrients</u> is emerging.

本句 evidence 后面紧跟着一个同位语从句，谓语很短，可将同位语从句移至句尾，达到句子平衡的效果。

译文 2　Evidence is emerging <u>that plant fibers have profound influences on human nutrition because they alter the absorption and metabolism of many nutrients</u>.

当一个句子的主语为不定式短语时，可将主语后移，句首用 it 做形式主语，从而使句子的结构变得匀称，并且也可使后移的主语得到强调。

Task 11　**Put the attributes of the following sentences in the right position to make the sentences balanced.**

1. Patients with oral lesions of this kind unassociated with gut lesions have also been described.

_____

2. Two patients who have presented with the characteristics of methane poisoning-metabolic acidosis and ocular toxicity have been studied.

3. A family in which three middle-aged siblings had unexplained cirrhosis and steatosis was studied.

4. After an X-ray examination, the question whether this patient should undergo an operation immediately arose.

5. To construct protoplasm in the lab has been attempted many times.

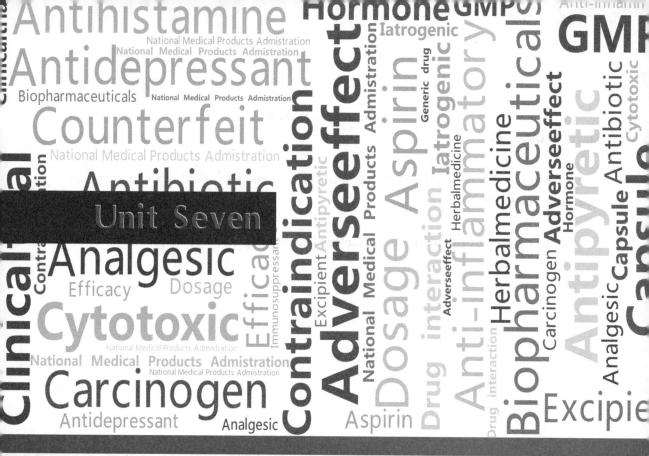

Unit Seven

Pharmacology

✓课文音频
✓听力音频
✓在线课程
✓课件申请

Receptors

Pharmacology is concerned with all facets of the interaction of chemicals with biological systems. When such interactions are applied to the cure or amelioration of disease, the chemicals are usually called drugs.

Most drugs produce effects by combining with biological receptors. The chemical bonds that form between drug molecule and receptor are usually reversible. The ease with which drug and receptor interact is influenced by the degree of complementarity of their respective three-dimensional structures. For this reason, minor chemical modification of a drug may produce profound changes in its pharmacological activity.

Pharmacology is a hybrid science. It freely draws upon the intellectual resources of all the basic medical sciences and contributes to every aspect of clinical medicine. It is appropriate, therefore, that the concept of receptors, a central theorem of pharmacology, should have arisen from the work of John Newport Langley, a physiologist, and Paul Ehrlich, a polymath best remembered for his work in immunology and in the chemotherapy of syphilis.

While still an undergraduate in the department of physiology at Cambridge University, Langley studied the antagonism by atropine of the contractile effects of pilocarpine on smooth muscle. Describing his results in 1878, he made the assumption "that there is a substance or substances in the nerve endings or gland cells with which both atropine and pilocarpine are capable of forming compounds. On this assumption then the atropine and pilocarpine compounds are formed according to some law of which their relative mass and

pharmacology /ˌfɑːməˈkɒlədʒi/ n. 药物学,药理学

amelioration /əˌmiːliəˈreɪʃən/ n. 改善,改良,改进

receptor /rɪˈseptə/ n. 感受器,受体

complementarity /ˌkɒmplɪmenˈtærɪti/ n. 补充,互补性
three-dimensional /ˌθriːdaɪˈmenʃənəl/ adj. 三维的
modification /ˌmɒdɪfɪˈkeɪʃən/ n. 修改,修正
pharmacological /ˌfɑːməkəˈlɒdʒɪkəl/ adj. 药物学的,药理学的
hybrid /ˈhaɪbrɪd/ n. 混合体,混合物
theorem /ˈθɪərəm/ n. 定理

polymath /ˈpɒlɪmæθ/ n. 博学的人

syphilis /ˈsɪfɪlɪs/ n. 梅毒

antagonism /ænˈtæɡəˌnɪzəm/ n. 对抗,对立,拮抗
atropine /ˈætrəupiːn/ n. 阿托品
contractile /kənˈtræktaɪl/ adj. 可收缩的,有收缩性的
pilocarpine /ˌpaɪləˈkɑːpiːn/ n. 匹鲁卡品,毛果芸香碱

chemical affinity for the substance are factors."

Over the next three decades a clearer picture of the nature of these "substances" evolved slowly in Langley's mind. Based upon his experiments with isolated nerve-muscle preparations, he concluded that the drug did not act directly on the nerve endings or on the muscle. He observed that nicotine causes contraction of muscle whether or not the muscle is innervated. Furthermore, curare, a drug then commonly thought to act upon nerve endings, blocks the effects of nicotine even in denervated muscle. Finally, a muscle paralyzed by curare still contracts when stimulated electrically. Langley concluded that nicotine and curare must combine with something that is neither nerve nor muscle; in 1905 he called it "receptive substance".

The subject of Ehrlich's M.D. thesis in 1878 was the histological utility of certain vital dyes. Impressed by the specificity with which dyes interact with tissues, he postulated that a drug can have a therapeutic effect only if it has "the right sort of affinity." However, his first application of this idea was to immunology rather than to pharmacology. In his side-chain theory, Ehrlich suggested that there is binding between toxins and antitoxins via chemically specific functional groups. Later he expanded this idea to include chemoreceptors located in parasites; these receptors could serve as targets for chemically aimed "magic bullet". Despite the appeal that such ideas have for modern pharmacologists, Ehrlich long resisted the application of his theory to drug-tissue interactions in general. There was simply too great a conceptual gap between the firm binding of an arsenical poison to a trypanosome and the evanescent effects of many drugs. But the passage of time, the accumulation of data, and in particular, a careful consideration of Langley's experiments eventually caused Ehrlich's "doubts to disappear and made the existence of chemoreceptors seem probable".

Today receptor theory serves as a unifying concept of the explanation of the effects of chemicals on

innervate /ɪˈnɜːveɪt/ vt. 分布神经，刺激

denervate /diːˈnɜːveɪt/ v. 除神经支配，去神经

paralyze /ˈpærəlaɪz/ vt. 使……瘫痪

curare /kjʊˈrɑːri/ n. [植]箭毒

postulate /ˈpɒstjʊleɪt/ vt. 要求，假定

chemoreceptor /ˈkiːməʊrɪseptə/ n. 化学受体，化学感应器

arsenical /ɑːˈsenɪkəl/ adj. 砷的

trypanosome /ˈtrɪpənəˌsəʊm/ n. 锥体虫

evanescent /ˌevəˈnesənt/ adj. 逐渐消失的

biological systems, whether these chemicals be of exogenous (pharmacological) or endogenous (physiological) origin. A modern statement of the receptor theorem is that of Goldstein, Aronow, and Kalman: in general, a drug produces a particular effect by combining chemically with some specific molecular constituent (receptor) of the biological system upon which it acts. The function of the receptor molecule in the biological system is thereby modified to produce a measurable effect.

exogenous /ek'sɒdʒənəs/ *adj.* 外生的，外源的，由外生长的
endogenous /en'dɒdʒənəs/ *adj.* 内生的，内源的

Task 1 **Find out the answers to the following questions and then compare your answers with a partner.**

1. Why could the minor chemical modification of a drug produce great change in its pharmacological activity?

2. Why does the author say pharmacology is a hybrid science?

3. How did Langley discover the receptive substance?

4. When can a drug have a therapeutic effect?

5. What is the modern statement of the receptor theorem?

Part II Listening

Task 2 **You will hear 20 words or phrases which will be read three times. Write them down on the blanks and check with your partner after you finish.**

1. _____ 2. _____ 3. _____ 4. _____

5. _____ 6. _____ 7. _____ 8. _____

9. _____ 10. _____ 11. _____ 12. _____

13. _____ 14. _____ 15. _____ 16. _____

17. _____ 18. _____ 19. _____ 20. _____

Task 3 You are going to hear a passage which will be read three times. Take some notes while you are listening to the passage and then answer the following questions.

1. What is the misunderstanding of drug addiction?

_____

2. What is the consequence of repeated drug use?

_____

3. What is the key to the treatment of drug addiction?

_____

Part Ⅲ   Oral Presentation and Discussion

Task 4 Read the following passage and make an oral presentation.

The Challenge of Rare Diseases —From Drug Development to Approval

Despite the approximately 7,000 rare diseases that affect millions of people worldwide, there are comparatively few treatments on the market. In addition to the issues pertaining to small markets, drug development for rare diseases poses unique scientific and ethical challenges.

The patient population affected by rare diseases is typically small, heterogeneous, and widely dispersed, complicating study enrollment, design, and replication. In many countries, there are few specialized sites that provide treatment and could serve as study sites, leading to difficulty acquiring large amounts of high-quality patient data. Additional difficulties arise from the frequently progressive, life-limiting or -threatening nature of rare diseases and the fact that over 50% of those affected by rare diseases are children. There are special ethical considerations for children participating in rare disease clinical trials that need to be anticipated. These are just some of the impediments slowing down the development and approval of life-saving orphan drugs.

New approaches in orphan drug development may offer valuable solutions to overcome these hurdles, streamlining both clinical trials and approval processes to bring much-needed treatments to the market more quickly. Here, we briefly outline some of these new approaches and how they differ from traditional practices.

Clinical Trials Adapted to Fit Small Study Populations

Rare drug trials are often hampered by poorly developed study endpoints, insufficient patient data, and inappropriate control groups. In orphan drug development in particular, efficient study designs with appropriate comparators are key to generating interpretable clinical data for approval. Designing efficient rare disease clinical trials with clinically meaningful endpoints, however, requires close collaboration among statisticians, clinicians, and other clinical trial professionals, and a strong focus on patient needs.

Identifying patients' most critical needs, for example, helps define novel endpoints that are focused, meaningful, and achieved more quickly. But even when endpoints are well-defined, rare disease clinical trials may not generate the amount and quality of data that would help speed up the approval process. Global clinical studies, novel uses of comparator arms, and trial enrichment strategies may offer tractable solutions when small patient populations make enrollment and clinical trial design challenging.

Study designs that follow various trial enrichment strategies, such as prognostic and predictive enrichment, can significantly reduce the heterogeneity of the patient population and avoid large variation in study outcomes:

• Prognostic enrichment reduces variability in disease progression rates by identifying high-risk subjects more likely to experience poor study outcomes.

• Predictive enrichment selects subjects more likely to respond to the candidate treatment based on genetic or other markers, supporting smaller trial sizes.

Rare disease drug development plans that include patients that don't meet the narrowly defined enrichment trial criteria into other parts of the development program can enhance their supportive data and safety database while improving their enrollment and retention.

Natural history studies can be used in novel ways to address control group issues and increase the statistical power of rare disease clinical studies. For example, Bayesian methods could be used to borrow information from a natural history study to improve the power of a small placebo group. Clinical sites in different regions could follow natural history study master protocols to uniformly collect verifiable patient data that could serve as external controls in future clinical trials. Prospective collection of case histories in parallel to the drug trial may be more robust than natural history data from older sources and shorten developmental time for new drugs.

If chosen carefully, rare disease study designs can additionally benefit from methods commonly used in regular clinical trials. Adaptive enrichment trial designs, for example, may help reveal orphan drug effects more efficiently and tailor either sample size or patient population.

Approval Flexibility and Expedited Programs

Although a special regulatory pathway for orphan drug development does not exist in the US, different expedited approval processes such as Fast Track, Breakthrough Therapy, Priority Review, and the Regenerative Medicine Advanced Therapy Designation are already in place for medicines addressing serious unmet patient needs.

Rare disease drugs often meet the designation requirements and may then receive an expedited approval. Breakthrough and Regenerative Medicine Advanced Therapy designation rely on preliminary clinical evidence demonstrating substantial improvement and lead to more frequent meetings with the sponsor and shortened (priority) review. Fast Track designation relies on clinical or nonclinical data and additionally provides increased guidance and rolling submissions of marketing applications.

Furthermore, current regulations provide flexibility with the kind and quantity of data deemed necessary in the case of less common diseases. A rare disease drug may be approved based on just one appropriately controlled trial as long as the trial provides sufficient evidence and safety information to allow for benefit/risk assessments. In some cases, the FDA even accepts non-traditional data on treatment effectiveness. For example, the FDA recently accepted in vitro data to bridge the approval of a marketing supplement for treatment of patients with certain mutations in the cystic fibrosis (CF) transmembrane conductance regulator (CFTR) gene. The approved therapy had previously been shown to be effective in CF patients with other specific gene mutations, and increased the treatable CF patients from 8% to 11%, including very small groups of patients affected by several mutations. Additionally, the FDA allows pre-approval access to promising treatments through the expanded access program.

Conclusion

Rare diseases pose broad challenges of clinical research, patient recruitment, and long development timelines. As of 2010, only about 200 of the roughly 7,000 officially designated rare diseases were treatable. Fortunately, the number of diseases with available therapies is increasing. Worldwide, there are a large number of development programs for drugs targeting a wide range of rare diseases. Sponsors should be diligent in investigating potentially innovative approaches to orphan drug development to ensure an efficient and effective design that supports this upward trend.

Task 5 **Theme-related discussion.**

Clinical trials are research studies that test a medical, surgical, or behavioral intervention among people. These trials are the primary ways that researchers determine if a new form of treatment or prevention, such as a new drug, diet, or medical device, is safe and effective among people. However, the small population of patients with rare diseases can make conducting clinical trials for orphan drugs difficult.

Please watch the MOOC, think about it, and discuss the following questions with your partner.

1. What are the ethical principles in using human subjects in clinical trials for drug development?

2. What are some new approaches to clinical trials for orphan drugs?

Part Ⅳ　Word Formation

drug［英］药

  pharmaco-［希］药

    pharmacodiagnosis /ˌfɑːməkəʊˌdaɪəɡ'nəʊsɪs/ *n*.药物诊断

    pharmacodynamic /ˌfɑːməkəʊdaɪ'næmɪk/ *adj*.药效的

    pharmacopeia /ˌfɑːməkəʊ'piːə/ *n*.处方汇编；药典

many［英］多

  poly-［希］多，多数

    polyclonal /ˌpɒlɪ'kləʊnəl/ *adj*.多细胞的

    polyase /'pɒlɪeɪs/ *n*.多糖酶，聚合酶

    polycythemia /ˌpɒlɪsaɪ'θiːmɪə/ *n*.红细胞增多症

round［英］围绕，环绕地

  para-［希］旁，周；近似

    paranephric /ˌpærə'nefrɪk/ *adj*.肾旁的

    parahepatic /ˌpærəhi'pætɪk/ *adj*.肝旁的

    paracystitis /ˌpærəsɪs'taɪtɪs/ *n*.膀胱周炎

inside［英］里面，内部

  end(o)- 内，内膜

    endometry /en'dɒmɪtri/ *n*.内腔容积测定法

    endothelium /ˌendəʊ'θiːlɪəm/ *n*.内皮

    endotoxin /ˌendəʊ'tɒksɪn/ *n*.内毒素

cerebral ganglion［英］丘脑

  thalam(o)-［希］丘脑

    thalamocortical /ˌθæləməʊ'kɔːtɪkəl/ *adj*.丘脑皮质的

    thalamomammillary /ˌθæləməʊ'mæmɪləri/ *adj*.丘脑乳头体的

    thalamotomy /ˌθælə'mɒtəmi/ *n*.丘脑切开术

over［英］上

  epi-［希］上

    eparterial /ˌepɑː'tɪərɪəl/ *adj*.动脉上的

    epithelial /ˌepɪ'θiːlɪəl/ *adj*.上皮的；皮膜的

    epidermitis /ˌepɪdə'maɪtɪs/ *n*.表皮炎

Task 6 Match each of the following terms with its definition.

1	endogenic	A	a loss or impairment of movement or sensation in a body part
2	paralysis	B	situated upon or above an artery
3	pharmacokinetics	C	derived or occurring internally
4	eparterial	D	surgical excision of a portion of the thalamus
5	polyneuropathy	E	the study of the action of drugs in the body
6	thalamotomy	F	a neurological condition involving pathological damage to the peripheral nerves

Task 7 Fill in the blanks with words or phrases given in the box. Change the form where necessary.

endometrium	pharmaceutical	paralyse	polycythemia
paramedic	polypeptide	thalamus	epiderm
epithelium	endocrine		

1. To know what a _____ is, it is best to break it down into its smallest components—amino acids.

2. The _____ system is a network of glands that produce and release hormones that control many body functions.

3. The effect of the drug is to _____ the nerves in the leg before the operation.

4. The new cancer drug is undergoing rigorous _____ regulation before it can be marketed.

5. The _____, also known as the mucosal layer or membrane, is the innermost layer of the uterus.

6. The _____ is a small structure within the brain located just above the brain stem between the cerebral cortex and the midbrain and has extensive nerve connections to both.

7. When the _____ is composed of a single layer of cells, it is called simple epithelial tissue.

8. Erythrocytosis, or _____, is a condition characterized by an increase in red blood cells.

9. In healthy individuals, restoration of a functional _____ barrier is highly efficient, whereas repair of the deeper dermal layer is less perfect.

10. A _____ provides emergency medical care to individuals in critical or life-threatening situations.

Part V Fast Reading

CDER Takes Measures to Tackle Stimulant Use Disorder

The Center for Drug Evaluation and Research (CDER) performs an essential public health task by making sure that safe and effective drugs are available to improve the health of people in the United States.

As part of the U. S. Food and Drug Administration (FDA), CDER regulates over-the-counter and prescription drugs, including biological therapeutics and generic drugs. This work covers more than just medicines. For example, fluoride toothpaste, antiperspirants, dandruff shampoos and sunscreens are all considered drugs.

Introduction

Stimulants can be approved prescription medications or illegal drugs, such as cocaine and methamphetamine, that speed up bodily systems and make people feel more awake, alert, or energetic. Prescription stimulants, such as Adderall (amphetamine/dextroamphetamine), Ritalin and Concerta (methylphenidate), or Vyvanse (lisdexamfetamine dimesylate), can be used to treat attention-deficient hyperactivity disorder (ADHD), binge-eating disorder, and narcolepsy (uncontrollable episodes of deep sleep), among other conditions. These medications can help manage symptoms such as short attention span and impulsive behavior.

Misuse of prescription stimulants and use of illegal stimulants can give rise to stimulant use disorder. Stimulant use disorder is a pattern of stimulant drug use that causes clinically significant impairment or distress. It can lead to dire health consequences, such as psychiatric problems, seizures, coma, and death.

Unfortunately, overdose fatalities involving stimulants have been increasing every year for over a decade, according to National Institutes of Health analyses of data collected by the Centers for Disease Control and Prevention (CDC). Drug overdose deaths involving cocaine rose steadily from nearly 7,000 in 2015 to almost 16,000 in 2019. From 2019 to 2021, cocaine-involved deaths increased by 54% to over 24,000 deaths. Drug overdose deaths involving other stimulants, primarily methamphetamine, rose from approximately 550 in 1999 to almost 24,000 in 2020, and continued to increase to just under 33,000 deaths in 2021. Many of these stimulant-involved deaths also involved high-potency synthetic opioids, primarily fentanyl.

Overdose fatality rates were generally higher for racial and ethnic minority groups, according to the CDC, with non-Hispanic Black individuals and American Indian/Alaska Native individuals experiencing the highest death rates for overdoses involving cocaine and overdoses involving stimulants other than cocaine, respectively, in 2019.

CDER's Response

Given the severity of this public health crisis, CDER has been working with other interested parties on ways to facilitate the development of treatments for stimulant use disorder. We recently published a draft guidance on developing drug treatments for this disorder. As of now, there are no effective medications to treat stimulant use disorder. Drug development is challenging because the disorder is heterogenous, meaning it can involve the use of different types of stimulants in different settings and for different reasons. Finding a medication to treat all patients, or even a subset of patients, with stimulant use disorder is difficult.

The draft guidance provides recommendations for early phase drug development, such as ensuring there are no adverse interactions between the investigational therapy and a stimulant, as it is possible (even likely) that a study participant may be taking both drugs simultaneously.

The draft guidance discusses the benefits and limitations of different methods to assess treatment response, such as biological testing (e.g., testing of urine and other body fluids), patient self-reporting, and capturing periods of non-use. The guidance also describes endpoints that sponsors may consider, including change in pattern of stimulant use and change in disease status using diagnostic criteria, as well as clinical outcome assessments (outcome measures that evaluate how patients feel or function) and changes in mortality and hospitalization rates among people with stimulant use disorder.

We believe this guidance will help pave the way for new drugs to treat stimulant use disorder, and we encourage interested parties to review the draft and provide comment by December 4, 2023.

CDER Updates Warnings to Improve Safe Use of Stimulants

Prescription stimulants can play a role in treating various disorders. They are the most common type of medication to treat ADHD and are also used as therapies for binge-eating disorder and narcolepsy. However, the use of prescription stimulants can lead to misuse and abuse (also called nonmedical use), which can result in addiction, overdose, and death. Therefore, sharing prescription stimulants with people for whom these medications are not prescribed and using one's prescription stimulant differently than prescribed are serious concerns.

To encourage the safe use of prescription stimulants, CDER announced in May 2023 that it will require changes to all medication labels in this drug class. We are mandating that sponsors add information to the prescribing information that patients should never share their prescription stimulants with anyone. In addition, the Boxed Warning, FDA's most prominent warning, will describe the risks of misuse, abuse, addiction, and overdose consistently across all prescription stimulant labels. The Boxed Warning will also advise health care professionals to monitor patients closely for signs and symptoms of misuse.

Connection to FDA's Overdose Prevention Framework

Understanding Drug Overdoses and Deaths

The drug overdose epidemic continues to worsen in the United States. Drug overdoses, both fatal and nonfatal, continue to impact our nation. Overdose deaths remain a leading cause of injury-related death in the United States. The majority of overdose deaths involve opioids. Deaths involving synthetic opioids (largely illicitly made fentanyl) and stimulants (such as cocaine and methamphetamine) have increased in recent years.

For every drug overdose that results in death, there are many more nonfatal overdoses, each one with its own emotional and economic toll. This fast-moving epidemic does not distinguish among age, sex, or state or county lines. People who have had at least one overdose are more likely to have another. If a person who has had an overdose is seen in the ED, there is an opportunity to help prevent a repeat overdose by linking an individual to care that can improve their health outcomes.

Timely data help improve coordination and promote readiness among health departments, community members, healthcare providers, public health, law enforcement, and government agencies, for regional or multiple state overdose increases.

FDA's Overdose Prevention Framework

Illicitly manufactured fentanyl, heroin, cocaine, or methamphetamine (alone or in combination) were involved in nearly 85% of drug overdose deaths in 24 states and the District of Columbia during January—June 2019. More than 3 out of 5 overdose deaths had at least one potential opportunity to link people to care before the fatal overdose or to implement life-saving actions when the fatal overdose occurred.

Drug overdose deaths can be prevented. CDC is working to prevent overdoses and substance use-related harms with the following strategies. Monitor, analyze, and communicate trends, build state, tribal, local, and territorial capacity, support providers, health systems, payors, and employers, partner with public safety and community organizations, raise public awareness and reduce stigma.

Connection to FDA's Overdose Prevention Framework

Our efforts on curbing stimulant abuse—through drug development for stimulant use disorder and through fostering safe use of prescription stimulants—align with FDA's initiatives to prevent overdose, known as the FDA Overdose Prevention Framework. As we continue to fight stimulant use disorder, the lessons we learn can and will be incorporated into the larger framework. Drug overdose has terrible and sometimes irreversible consequences for many people, and our agency is working hard to address this public health crisis.

Task 8 Read the passage and decide whether the statements are true or false. If it is true, write "T". If it is not, write "F".

1. As a part of the U. S. Food and Drug Administration (FDA), CDER regulates over-the-counter and prescription drugs, excluding antiperspirants, dandruff shampoos and sunscreens. ( )

2. Drug overdose deaths involving other stimulants, primarily cocaine, rose from approximately 550 in 1999 to almost 24,000 in 2020. ( )

3. Stimulant use disorder is a pattern of stimulant drug use that causes clinically significant impairment or distress, and there are no effective medications to treat stimulant use disorder. ( )

4. The use of prescription stimulants can lead to misuse and abuse (also called nonmedical use), which can result in addiction, overdose, and death. ( )

5. Developing drugs for stimulant use disorder and fostering the safe use of prescription stimulants are aligned with the FDA Overdose Prevention Framework.
( )

Task 9 Please read the passage again and write a two-hundred-word synopsis.

Part Ⅵ Translation

Task 10 Please analyze the following sentences and then put them into Chinese.

1. Pharmacology is concerned with all facets of the interaction of chemicals with biological systems. Most drugs produce effects by combining with biological receptors.

_____

_____

2. Pharmacology is a hybrid science. It freely draws upon the intellectual resources of all the basic medical sciences and contributes to every aspect of clinical medicine.

_____

_____

3. Today receptor theory serves as a unifying concept of the explanation of the effects of chemicals on biological systems, whether these chemicals be of exogenous

(pharmacological) or endogenous (physiological) origin.

同位语

同位语是由两个或两个以上同一层次语法单位组成的结构,其中前项和后项所指相同,句法功能也相同,属于后置修饰语。同位语的结构、形式和作用是大家所熟悉的内容,在此不赘述。本节主要讨论同位语在汉英翻译和写作中的用法。

好文章的标准之一是简洁、清晰。就文风而言,应该用尽可能少的文字表达尽可能多而复杂的意思。同位语可以把句中所有处于从属地位的修饰语都聚集在关键和核心信息的周围,从而使句子的重点突出。

例1 更小血管在皮髓质结合处成为竖支,被称作弓状动脉。

译文1 The smaller arteries provide perpendicular branches at the corticomedullary junction known as the arcuate arteries.

译文2 The smaller arteries provide perpendicular branches, the arcuate arteries, at the corticomedullary junction.

例2 米歇尔·罗奇今年34岁,是加利福尼亚的一个国际法学家,像许多寻找更健康的生活方式的人一样,她开始求助于天然药物。

译文1 Michelle Roche is 34. She is a California publicist. Like many people looking for a more healthful life-style, she has turned to natural remedies.

译文2 Like many people looking for a more healthful life-style, Michelle Roche, 34, a California publicist, has turned to natural remedies.

以上例句的译文2均用同位语表达,比译文1的表达简洁明了。

例3 随着年龄的变化,弹性蛋白变粗,碎片化,需要获得更大的钙亲和力,这有可能造成动脉粥样硬化。

Elastin thickens, fragments, and acquires a greater affinity for calcium with age — changes that may also be associated with the development of antherosclerosis.

例4 葡萄糖在肌体中是最丰富的糖类,它在衰老的过程中也可能起作用。

Glucose, the most abundant sugar in the body, may play a role in the aging process.

例5 病理学的最终目的在于确定疾病的原因,从而达到防治疾病的目标。

The ultimate goal of pathology is the identification of the causes of disease, a fundamental objective that leads the way to disease prevention.

Task 11 **Translate the following sentences into Chinese.**

1. 她心率急剧上升，且伴有打嗝，这是一个危险的征兆，说明她的体内压力太大了。

_____

2. 这些肌肉通过收缩，也就是牵拉进行工作。

_____

3. 出现单独一个症状，如短期内体重减轻，就需要立即进行身体检查。

_____

4. 我们得出的一个结论是这些细胞在免疫反应中起着重要作用。

_____

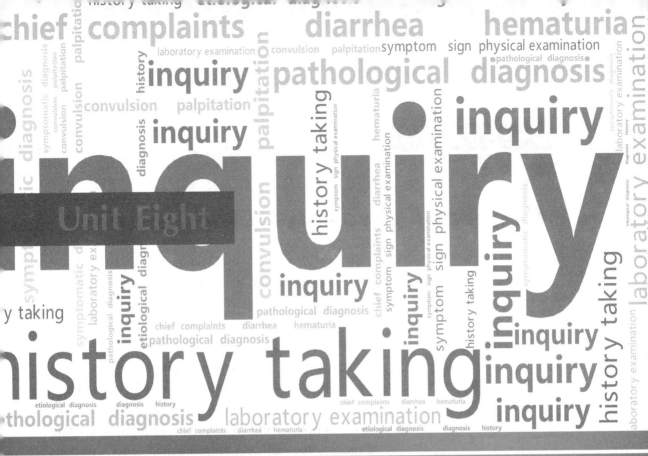

Diagnostics

✓课文音频
✓听力音频
✓在线课程
✓课件申请

General Approach to the Patient

familial /fəˈmɪliəl/ *adj.* 家族的，家族遗传的

Successful diagnosis and treatment demand that the practitioners consider the often complex personal, familial, and economic circumstances of the patient and establish and maintain a supportive and open relationship.

pertinent /ˈpɜːtɪnənt/ *adj.* 相关的
susceptible /səˈseptəbl/ *adj.* 易受外界影响的，易受感染的
commission /kəˈmɪʃən/ *n.* 委托，委任

The approach to diagnosis begins with the history and pertinent physical examination, each of which is susceptible to errors of omission and commission. The medical interview should accomplish three important functions: to collect information, to respond appropriately to the patient's emotional state, and to educate the patient and beneficially influence patient behavior. Patient satisfaction may be increased by discussion of psychosocial issues and by forgoing physician dominance of the encounter. If diagnostic procedures are indicated, they must be based on principles of diagnostic test selection which in turn depend upon the test characteristics (sensitivity and specificity), the disease incidence and prevalence, the potential risk to the patient, and the cost-benefit profile of the test determined by reference to the indications for it. Successful treatment—particularly management of patients with chronic illness—must be tailored to the circumstances of the individual patient and reinforced by a well-established doctor-patient relationship.

profile /ˈprəʊfaɪl/ *n.* 侧面，轮廓；图表，图谱
indication /ˌɪndɪˈkeɪʃən/ *n.* 指征，适应证
tailor /ˈteɪlə/ *vt.* 调整，使适合
reinforce /ˌriːɪnˈfɔːs/ *vt.* 加固，加强，增强

Guiding Principles

ethical /ˈeθɪkəl/ *adj.* 伦理的，道德的
undergird /ˌʌndəˈɡɜːd/ *vt.* 从底层加固，加强
beneficence /bɪˈnefɪsəns/ *n.* 仁慈，善行

Fundamental ethical principles must also undergird a successful approach to diagnosis and treatment: honesty, beneficence, justice, avoidance of conflict of interest, and the pledge to do no harm. Increasingly, Western medicine has involved patients in important decisions about medical care, including how far to proceed with treatment of patients with terminal illness.

Finally, the physician's role does not end with diagnosis and the prescribing of a treatment regimen. The importance of the empathic physician in helping patients and their families bear the burden of serious illness and death cannot be overemphasized. "To cure sometimes, to relieve often, and to comfort always" is a French saying as apt today as it was five centuries ago—as is Francis Peabody's admonition: "The secret of the care of the patient is in caring for the patient."

empathic /emˈpæθɪk/ adj. 移情作用的,感情移入的,共情的

admonition /ˌædməˈnɪʃən/ n. 警告,劝告

Health Maintenance and Disease Prevention

Preventing disease is more important than treating it. Preventive medicine is categorized as primary, secondary, or tertiary. Primary prevention aims to remove or reduce disease risk factors (e. g., immunization, giving up or not starting smoking). Secondary prevention techniques promote early detection of disease or precursor states (e. g., routine cervical Papanicolaou screening to detect invasive carcinoma or carcinoma in situ of the cervix, or tuberculin skin testing to identify candidates for chemoprophylaxis of tuberculosis). Tertiary prevention measures are aimed at limiting the impact of established disease (e. g., partial mastectomy and radiation therapy to remove and control localized breast cancer). Primary prevention is by far the most effective and economical of all methods of disease control, but most physicians are deficient in their counseling practices concerning preventable conditions.

tertiary /ˈtɜːʃəri/ adj. 第三的,第三位的

Papanicolaou /ˌpæpəˌnɪkəʊˈleɪuː/ 帕帕尼古拉乌(希腊医师和解剖学家)
in situ /ɪn ˈsaɪtjuː/ adj. 原位的
cervix /ˈsɜːvɪks/ n. 颈部,子宫颈
tuberculin /tjuːˈbɜːkjuːlɪn/ n. 结核菌素
chemoprophylaxis /ˌkeməʊˌprɒfiˈlæksɪs/ n. 化学预防,化学品预防
tuberculosis /tjuːˌbɜːkjʊˈləʊsɪs/ n. 肺结核
mastectomy /mæsˈtektəmi/ n. 乳房切除术

Physicians can have a major role in reducing almost all of the risk factors. Health maintenance and disease prevention usually begin with the office or clinic encounter.

Physical Inactivity and Sedentary Life-style

A sedentary life-style has been linked to 28% of deaths from leading chronic disease. Physical inactivity is a major risk factor for heart disease.

The Centers for Disease Control and Prevention recently recommended that every adult should accumulate 30 minutes or more of moderate-intensity physical activity on most, preferably all, days of the week. The new guideline is intended to complement, not replace, previous advice urging at least 20—30 minutes of more vigorous, continuous aerobic exercise three to five times a week.

Regular moderate to vigorous exercise has been shown to lower the risk of myocardial infarction, stroke, hypertension, type Ⅱ diabetes mellitus, diverticular disease, and osteoporosis. In general, the benefits of exercise appear to be dose-dependent, with a major difference in benefit between no and mild to moderate exercise and a smaller difference in benefit between moderate and vigorous exercise. In recent studies, the relative risk of stroke was found to be less than one-sixth in men who exercised vigorously compared with those who were inactive; the relative risk of non-insulin-dependent diabetes mellitus was about half among men who exercised five or more times weekly compared with those who exercised once a week. Glucose control is improved in diabetics who exercise regularly, even at a modest level. Regular exercise is associated with a lower long-term risk of coronary events, including fatal myocardial infarctions, with elevated HDL, cholesterol concentrations in both men and women and with decreased risk of hypertension. Physical activity reduces the risk of colon cancer (though not rectal cancer) in men and women and of breast and reproductive organ cancer in women. Finally weight-bearing exercise has been shown to increase bone mineral content and retard development of osteoporosis in women.

diabetes /ˌdaɪəˈbiːtiːz/
mellitus /məˈlaɪtəs/ 糖尿病
diverticular /ˌdaɪvəˈtɪkjʊlə/ adj. 憩室的,膨部的
osteoporosis /ˌɒstiəʊpəˈrəʊsɪs/ n. 骨质疏松症
dose-dependent adj. 取决于剂量的

non-insulin-dependent adj. 非胰岛素依赖型的

colon /ˈkəʊlən/ n. 结肠
rectal /ˈrektəl/ adj. 直肠的

retard /rɪˈtɑːd/ n. 迟延,减速

Task 1 Find out the answers to the following questions and then compare your answers with a partner.

1. What are susceptible to errors of omission and commission in making diagnosis?

2. What do you think a qualified physician should do to come to successful diagnosis and treatment according to the text?

3. Why has western medicine involved patients in important decisions about medical care?

4. Why does the author think physicians have a major role in primary prevention?

5. How many diseases the author mentions in the text can be preventable?

Part II Listening

Task 2 You will hear 20 words or phrases which will be read three times. Write them down on the blanks and check with your partner after you finish.

1. _____ 2. _____ 3. _____ 4. _____

5. _____ 6. _____ 7. _____ 8. _____

9. _____ 10. _____ 11. _____ 12. _____

13. _____ 14. _____ 15. _____ 16. _____

17. _____ 18. _____ 19. _____ 20. _____

Task 3 You are going to hear a passage which will be read three times. Take some notes while you are listening to the passage and then answer the following questions.

1. What is a misdiagnosis?

_____

2. What is a missed diagnosis?

_____

3. What can you do if you think your diagnosis is not correct?

_____

Task 4 Read the following passage and make an oral presentation.

Age and Chronic Illness on Life Expectancy after a Diagnosis of Colorectal Cancer

We found a strong relationship between chronic illness and life expectancy after cancer diagnosis. The relationship was strongest among patients who received a diagnosis of early-stage cancer. We also found substantial variation in life expectancy after a diagnosis of stage I colorectal cancer among older persons. Patients with several chronic conditions had a substantially lower gain in life expectancy associated with early-stage cancer at diagnosis than did their counterparts without such conditions. For instance, a 75-year-old woman with no chronic conditions had a life expectancy of more than 15 years after a stage I cancer diagnosis. If she had 3 or more conditions, however, her life expectancy was approximately 5 years and her benefit from screening would be marginal. This is because she would be unlikely to survive to the point (approximately 4 years) where, in clinical trials of screening, patients randomly assigned to screening had a lower colorectal cancer mortality rate than unscreened participants. These findings suggest that physicians must consider the burden of chronic illness in conjunction with age to estimate the benefits associated with an early diagnosis of colorectal cancer.

Although interest in targeting colorectal cancer screening efforts to patients who would benefit the most from early diagnosis has increased, whether current practices are consistent with these recommendations is unclear. We found that patients with a higher burden of chronic illness were just as likely to receive a diagnosis of stage Ⅰ cancer as those without such conditions. Further work should explore the effect of individualized data about screening risks and benefits on decision making. Targeting screening efforts to patients with a greater expected benefit is also important from a societal perspective. An estimated 40 million adults older than 50 years of age have not been screened for colorectal cancer. Endoscopic screening for all of them would take up to 10 years according to estimates of existing capacity. Given the limited colonoscopy resources, the distribution of resources to colorectal cancer screening, as well as screening guidelines and quality-of-care assessments, should take into account the expected benefits, which we have shown to depend on chronic disease burden.

Although the association with life expectancy can vary across chronic conditions, we found that incorporating specific conditions into life expectancy estimates can be challenging. Not only did the conditions we investigated frequently occur in combination, we also found that knowing a specific combination is clinically relevant. For instance, the life expectancy for an 81-year-old patient with diabetes and heart or vascular disease was about 5 years, which is in contrast to the 8-year life expectancy for a patient with diabetes alone and the 7-year life expectancy for a patient with heart or vascular disease alone. Therefore, a specific recommendation about screening patients with heart disease may not apply to all patients. While our approach to counting comorbid conditions corresponds well to population-based data, future work should explore how to integrate specific conditions and combinations of conditions into more precise estimates of life expectancy—a task that we have begun.

We also found that the burden of chronic conditions was strongly related to survival, regardless of whether patients had received adjuvant therapy. This suggests that chronic conditions exert a substantive effect on survival that is independent of their effect on decisions to give adjuvant therapy or its effectiveness. While several comorbid conditions may certainly alter a person's willingness to undergo cancer-specific therapy, our findings suggest that the main mechanism by which comorbid conditions affect life expectancy is through the competing causes of death attributable to these conditions. Therefore, even among patients who are willing to undergo cancer treatment, chronic condition status should inform screening decisions.

Our analyses have several limitations. Administrative claims underestimate the prevalence of many chronic conditions, such as dementia, and the burden of chronic conditions for many patients was probably higher than that noted in their administrative claims. In addition, patients vary in the incidence of additional conditions after cancer diagnosis, which would add heterogeneity to life expectancy estimates within the chronic illness groups. Furthermore, our analysis focused on death as the sole outcome of interest. Future work should incorporate self-reported chronic illness and health status data to derive more comprehensive assessments of quality-adjusted life expectancy, as well as nonfatal outcomes of interest. We derived our life expectancy estimates from a life-table method, and survival probabilities for individuals within each age or chronic condition group could vary substantially. However, although a specific person's length of life is impossible to predict with certainty, patients would benefit from understanding the probabilities of reaching selected outcomes and how these probabilities vary with different screening strategies. Future work should explore the effect of screening across different patient age and chronic illness groups, as well as the effect of repeated screening and the variation in the relative contribution of colorectal cancer and non-colorectal cancer death to outcomes. Our analysis of specific conditions, and their interactions, demonstrated that conditions do vary in how they affect patient outcomes.

Task 5 **Theme-related discussion.**

Diagnostics is the branch of medical science that deals with diagnosis. The methods of traditional Chinese diagnostics include visual, auditory, olfactory, tactile forms of observation and questioning, which are determined by the tremendous wisdom of "harmony" in Traditional Chinese Medicine, manifested in the harmony among all parts of the human body, between the human body and the spirit, and between man and nature.

Please watch the MOOC, think about it, and discuss the following questions with your partner.

1. How can the traditional Chinese diagnostics be introduced to foreigners?

2. What is the philosophy and mechanism behind acupuncture therapy?

Part Ⅳ Word Formation

neck〔英〕颈

cervic(o)-〔拉〕颈

    cervicitis /ˌsɜːvɪˈsaɪtɪs/ *n*. 宫颈炎

    cervicobrachial /ˌsɜːvɪkəʊˈbreɪkiəl/ *adj*. 颈臂的

    cervicodynia /ˌsɜːvɪkəʊˈdɪniə/ *n*. 颈痛

bone〔英〕骨

oste(o)-〔希〕骨

    osteoarthritis /ˌɒstɪəʊɑːˈθraɪtɪs/ *n*. 骨关节炎

    osteoporosis /ˌɒstɪəʊpəˈrəʊsɪs/ *n*. 骨质疏松

    osteoplast /ˈɒstɪəʊplæst/ *n*. 成骨细胞

resect〔英〕切除

-ectomy〔希〕切除术

    adenectomy /ˌædɪˈnektəmi/ *n*. 腺切除术

    ovariectomy /əʊˌvɛərɪˈektəmi/ *n*. 卵巢切除术

    splenectomy /splɪˈnektəmi/ *n*. 脾切除术

illness〔英〕疾病

-osis〔希〕病,病态

    neurosis /njʊˈrəʊsɪs/ *n*. 神经官能症

    angiosclerosis /ˌændʒɪəʊskləˈrəʊsɪs/ *n*. 血管硬化

    myomatosis /ˌmaɪəʊməˈtəʊsɪs/ *n*. 肌瘤病

adrenal body〔英〕肾上腺

adren(o)-〔拉〕肾上腺

    adrenocortical /əˌdriːnəʊˈkɔːtɪkl/ *adj*. 肾上腺皮质的

    adrenocorticotropin /əˈdriːnəʊkɔːtɪkəʊˈtrɒpɪn/ *n*. 促皮质素,促肾上腺皮质激素

    adrenotoxin /əˌdriːnəʊˈtɒksɪn/ *n*. 肾上腺毒素

wound〔英〕创伤

traumat(o)-〔希〕创伤,外伤

    traumatology /ˌtrɔːməˈtɒlədʒi/ *n*. 创伤学

traumatonesis /ˌtrɔːməˈtəʊnəsɪs/ *n*. 创口缝术

traumatotherapy /ˌtrɔːmətəˈθerəpi/ *n*. 创伤性疗法

Task 6 **Match each of the following terms with its definition.**

1	angiostenosis	A	epinephrine, a type of hormone that is released whenever a person experiences fear, anxiety, or stress
2	cervicotomy	B	the narrowing of one or more blood vessels
3	adrenalin	C	a physician specializing in treating wounds and injuries caused by accidents or violence
4	osteitis	D	surgical removal of a kidney
5	nephrectomy	E	inflammation of bone or bony tissue
6	traumatologist	F	incision into the cervix of the uterus

Task 7 **Fill in the blanks with words or phrases given in the box. Change the form where necessary.**

adrenal gland	ovariectomy	trauma	cervix
adrenomedullary	osteomyelitis	cervicothoracic	osteopenia
sclerosis	traumatic shock		

1. The _____ are located in the posterior abdomen, between the superomedial kidney and the diaphragm.

2. When you have _____ , your bones are weaker than they used to be but not weak enough for you to be diagnosed with osteoporosis.

3. Multiple _____ is a disease that impacts the brain, spinal cord and optic nerves, which make up the central nervous system and controls everything we do.

4. Complex psychological _____ is more complicated and pervasive than isolated traumatic events, occurring mainly in vulnerable periods resulting in severe compromise of childhood development.

5. Common stimuli for the secretion of _____ hormones include exercise, hypoglycemia, hemorrhage, and emotional distress.

6. _____ is an intense emotional response to a deeply distressing or disturbing event, such as loss, abuse, or natural disaster.

7. _____ spine joint manipulation or mobilization is a physiotherapy or chiropractic intervention that can be used for neck, back or shoulder pain.

8. A person affected either with ovarian cancer or cysts, benign tumors, abscesses or pelvic infection, or ectopic pregnancy will be eligible for _____ .

9. A diagnosis of _____ should be considered in any patient with acute onset or progressive worsening of musculoskeletal pain accompanied by constitutional symptoms such as fever, malaise, lethargy, and irritability.

10. Inflammation of the neck of the womb, _____, can also be caused by other conditions.

Part V Fast Reading

Screening and Diagnosis of Autism Spectrum Disorder

What is Autism Spectrum Disorder?

Autism spectrum disorder (ASD) is a developmental disability caused by differences in the brain. Some people with ASD have a known difference, such as a genetic condition. Other causes are not yet known. Scientists believe there are multiple causes of ASD that act together to change the most common ways people develop. We still have much to learn about these causes and how they impact people with ASD.

People with ASD may behave, communicate, interact, and learn in ways that are different from most other people. There is often nothing about how they look that sets them apart from other people. The abilities of people with ASD can vary significantly. For example, some people with ASD may have advanced conversation skills whereas others may be nonverbal. Some people with ASD need a lot of help in their daily lives; others can work and live with little to no support.

ASD begins before the age of 3 years and can last throughout a person's life, although symptoms may improve over time. Some children show ASD symptoms within the first 12 months of life. In others, symptoms may not show up until 24 months of age or later. Some children with ASD gain new skills and meet developmental milestones until around 18 to 24 months of age, and then they stop gaining new skills or lose the skills they once had.

As children with ASD become adolescents and young adults, they may have difficulties developing and maintaining friendships, communicating with peers and adults, or understanding what behaviors are expected in school or on the job. They may come to the attention of healthcare providers because they also have conditions such as anxiety, depression, or attention-deficit/hyperactivity disorder, which occur more often in people with ASD than in people without ASD.

Diagnosis

Diagnosing ASD can be difficult because there is no medical test, like a blood test, to diagnose the disorder. Doctors look at the child's developmental history and behavior to make a diagnosis.

ASD can sometimes be detected at 18 months of age or younger. By age 2, a diagnosis by an experienced professional can be considered reliable. However, many children do not receive a final diagnosis until much older. Some people are not diagnosed until they are adolescents or adults. This delay means that people with ASD might not get the early help they need.

Diagnosing children with ASD as early as possible is important to make sure children receive the services and supports they need to reach their full potential.

Developmental Monitoring

Developmental monitoring is an active, ongoing process of watching a child grow and encouraging conversations between parents and providers about a child's skills and abilities. Developmental monitoring involves observing how your child grows and whether your child meets the typical developmental milestones, or skills that most children reach by a certain age, in playing, learning, speaking, behaving, and moving.

Parents, grandparents, early childhood education providers, and other caregivers can participate in developmental monitoring. CDC's "Learn the Signs. Act Early." program has developed free materials, including CDC's Milestone Tracker app, to help parents and providers work together to monitor your child's development and know when there might be a concern and if more screening is needed. You can use a brief checklist of milestones to see how your child is developing. If you notice that your child is not meeting milestones, talk with your doctor or nurse about your concerns and ask about developmental screening. Learn more about CDC Milestone Tracker app, milestone checklists, and other parent materials.

When you take your child to a well visit, your doctor or nurse will also do developmental monitoring. The doctor or nurse might ask you questions about your child's development or will talk and play with your child to see if they are developing and meeting milestones.

Your doctor or nurse may also ask about your child's family history. Be sure to let your doctor or nurse know about any conditions that your child's family members have, including ASD, learning disorders, intellectual disability, or attention deficit/hyperactivity disorder (ADHD).

Developmental Screening

Developmental screening takes a closer look at how your child is developing.

Developmental screening is more formal than developmental monitoring. It is a regular part of some well-child visits even if there is not a known concern.

The American Academy of Pediatrics (AAP) recommends developmental and behavioral screening for all children during regular well-child visits at these ages:

9 months

18 months

30 months

In addition, AAP recommends that all children be screened specifically for ASD during regular well-child visits at these ages:

18 months

24 months

Screening questionnaires and checklists are based on research that compares your child to other children of the same age. Questions may ask about language, movement, and thinking skills, as well as behaviors and emotions. Developmental screening can be done by a doctor or nurse, or other professionals in healthcare, community, or school settings. Your doctor may ask you to complete a questionnaire as part of the screening process.

Screening at times other than the recommended ages should be done if you or your doctor have a concern. Additional screening should also be done if a child is at high risk for ASD (for example, having a sibling or other family member with ASD) or if behaviors sometimes associated with ASD are present. If your child's healthcare provider does not periodically check your child with a developmental screening test, you can ask that it be done.

Developmental Diagnosis

A brief test using a screening tool does not provide a diagnosis, but it can indicate whether a child is on the right development track or if a specialist should take a closer look. If the screening tool identifies an area of concern, a formal developmental evaluation may be needed. This formal evaluation is a more in-depth look at a child's development and is usually done by a trained specialist such as a developmental pediatrician, child psychologist, speech-language pathologist, occupational therapist, or other specialist. The specialist may observe the child, give the child a structured test, ask the parents or caregivers questions, or ask them to fill out questionnaires. The results of this formal evaluation highlight your child's strengths and challenges and can inform whether they meet criteria for a developmental diagnosis.

A diagnosis of ASD now includes several conditions that used to be diagnosed separately: autistic disorder, pervasive developmental disorder not otherwise specified (PDD-NOS), and Asperger syndrome. Your doctor or other healthcare provider can help you understand and navigate the diagnostic process.

The results of a formal developmental evaluation can also inform whether your child needs early intervention services. In some cases, the specialist might recommend genetic counseling and testing for your child.

Task 8 **Read the passage and decide whether the statements are true or false. If it is true, write "T". If it is not, write "F".**

1. People with ASD may come to the attention of healthcare providers because they may have difficulties in communicating with peers.   (   )

2. Diagnosing ASD can be difficult because there is a lack of experienced professional doctors.   (   )

3. Developmental monitoring involves observing how your child grows and whether your child meets the typical developmental milestones, or skills.   (   )

4. AAP recommends that all children be screened specifically for ASD during regular well-child visits at 30 months.   (   )

5. The formal development evaluation is a more in-depth look at a child's development and is usually done by a trained specialist.   (   )

Task 9 **Read the passage again and write a two-hundred-word synopsis.**

Part Ⅵ Translation

Task 10 **Analyze the following sentences and then put them into Chinese.**

1. The new guideline is intended to complement, not replace, previous advice urging at least 20—30 minutes of more vigorous, continuous aerobic exercise three to five times a week.

_____

_____

2. In general, the benefits of exercise appear to be dose-dependent, with a major difference in benefit between no and mild to moderate exercise and a smaller difference in benefit between moderate and vigorous exercise.

_____

_____

3. Patients with several chronic conditions had a substantially lower gain in life expectancy associated with early-stage cancer at diagnosis than did their counterparts without such conditions.

_____

_____

医学翻译技巧

主谓一致

由于英汉两种语言表达上的差异,在翻译摘要或写作时,作者有时会写出一些主谓不一致的句子,特别是当主谓语之间有其他成分时,容易出现主谓不一致的现象。为了保证主谓一致,就要抓住句子的中心词。中心词是单数时,谓语动词要用第三人称单数形式;中心词是复数时,谓语动词要做相应变化。

例 1　**Animals** without any treatment <u>was</u> used as a normal control.

本句中的主语中心词是复数名词 animals,所以谓语应该使用 be 动词的复数形式 were。本句应修改为:

Animals without any treatment <u>were</u> used as a normal control.

例 2　Ten weeks later, oral glucose tolerance <u>test</u>(OGTT)<u>were</u> performed in all groups.

本句的主语中心词是单数名词 test,所以谓语应使用 be 动词的单数形式 was。本句应修改为:

Ten weeks later, oral glucose tolerance **test**(OGTT)<u>was</u> performed in all groups.

Task 11 **Translate the following sentences into English.**

1. 这些患者年龄在 40～60 岁之间。

_____

2. 本文报导了 5 例患者死亡。

_____

3. 类风湿关节炎的早期特征是时好时坏。

_____

4. 在敏感性、特异性和准确性上均有显著差异。

_____

5. 他是那些医生中唯一一位愿意动手术的医生。

_____

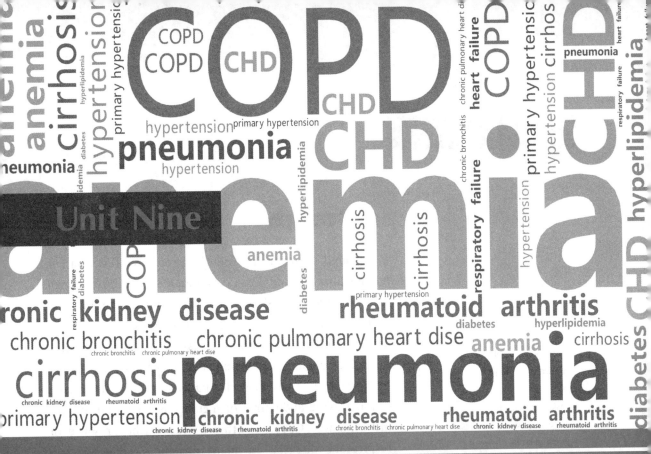

Unit Nine

Internal Medicine

✓课文音频
✓听力音频
✓在线课程
✓课件申请

Part I Text

Cough

Cough performs an essential protective function for human airways and lungs. Without an effective cough reflex, we are at risk for retained airway secretions and aspirated material predisposing to infection, atelectasis, and respiratory compromise. At the other extreme, excessive coughing can be exhausting; can be complicated by emesis, syncope, muscular pain, or rib fractures; and can aggravate abdominal or inguinal hernias and urinary incontinence. Cough is often a clue to the presence of respiratory disease. In many instances, cough is an expected and accepted manifestation of disease, as in acute respiratory tract infection. However, persistent cough in the absence of other respiratory symptoms commonly causes patients to seek medical attention.

Impaired Cough

Weak or ineffective cough compromises the ability to clear lower respiratory tract infections, predisposing to more serious infections and their sequelae. Weakness, paralysis, or pain of the expiratory (abdominal and intercostal) muscles is foremost on the list of causes of impaired cough (Table 1). A variety of assistive devices and techniques have been developed to improve cough strength, running the gamut from simple (splinting of the abdominal muscles with a tightly-held pillow to reduce postoperative pain while coughing) to complex (a mechanical cough-assist device supplied via face mask or tracheal tube that applies a cycle of positive pressure followed rapidly by negative pressure).

predispose /ˌpriːdɪˈspəʊz/ v. 易患某病,易感

atelectasis /ˌætəˈlektəsɪs/ n. 肺不张

complicate /ˈkɒmplɪkeɪt/ v. 并发疾病

emesis /ˈeməsɪs/ n. 呕吐

syncope /ˈsɪŋkəpi/ n. 晕厥

inguinal hernia /ˈɪŋgwɪnəl/ /ˈhɜːniə/ 腹股沟疝

sequelae /sɪˈkwiːlə/ (pl. sequelae) 后遗症

gamut /ˈgæmət/ n. 全域,全范围

Table 1 CAUSES OF IMPAIRED COUGH

Decreased expiratory-muscle strength

Decreased inspiratory-muscle strength

Chest wall deformity

Impaired glottic closure or tracheostomy

Tracheomalacia

Abnormal airway secretions

Central respiratory depression (e. g., anesthesia, sedation, or coma)

glottic /'glɒtɪk/ *adj.* 声门的
tracheomalacia /ˌtreɪkɪəmə'leɪʃɪə/ *n.* 气管软骨软化

Symptomatic Cough

The cough of chronic bronchitis in long-term cigarette smokers rarely leads the patient to seek medical advice. It lasts for only seconds to a few minutes, is productive of benign appearing mucoid sputum, and generally does not cause discomfort. Cough may occur in the context of other respiratory symptoms that together point to a diagnosis; for example, cough accompanied by wheezing, shortness of breath, and chest tightness after exposure to a cat or other sources of allergens suggests asthma. At times, however, cough is the dominant or sole symptom of disease, and it may be of sufficient duration and severity that relief is sought. The duration of cough is a clue to its etiology. Acute cough (<3 weeks) is most commonly due to a respiratory tract infection, aspiration, or inhalation of noxious chemicals or smoke. Subacute cough (3~8 weeks in duration) is a common residuum of tracheobronchitis, as in pertussis or "postviral tussive syndrome." Chronic cough (>8 weeks) may be caused by a wide variety of cardiopulmonary diseases, including those of inflammatory, infectious, neoplastic, and cardiovascular etiologies. When initial assessment with chest examination and radiography is normal, cough-variant asthma, gastroesophageal reflux, nasopharyngeal drainage, and medications (angiotensin-converting enzyme [ACE] inhibitors) are the most

sputum /'spjuːtəm/ *n.* 痰

asthma /'æsmə/ *n.* 哮喘

residuum /rɪ'zɪdjʊəm/ *n.* 残余,剩余
pertussis /pə'tʌsɪs/ *n.* 百日咳
tussive /'tʌsɪv/ *adj.* 咳嗽的

common causes of chronic cough.

Symptom-Based Treatment of Cough

idiopathic /ˌɪdɪəˈpæθɪk/ adj. 自发的，特发的

Chronic idiopathic cough, also called cough hypersensitivity syndrome, is distressingly common. It is often experienced as a tickle or sensitivity in the throat, occurs more often in women, and is typically "dry" or at most productive of scant amounts of mucoid sputum. It can be exhausting, interfere with work, and cause social embarrassment. Once serious underlying cardiopulmonary pathology has been excluded, an attempt at cough suppression is appropriate. Most effective are narcotic

narcotic /nɑːˈkɒtɪk/ adj. 麻醉的，镇静的

cough suppressants, such as codeine or hydrocodone, which are thought to act in the "cough center" in the brainstem. The tendency of narcotic cough suppressants to cause drowsiness and constipation and their potential for addictive dependence limit their appeal for long-term

dextromethorphan /ˌdekstrəʊmiˈθɔːfən/ n. 右美沙芬

use. Dextromethorphan is an over-the-counter, centrally acting cough suppressant with fewer side effects and less efficacy than the narcotic cough suppressants. Dextromethorphan is thought to have a different site of action than narcotic cough suppressants and can be used in combination with them if necessary. Benzonatate is

benzonatate /benˈzəʊnəteɪt/ n. 苯佐那酯

thought to inhibit neural activity of sensory nerves in the cough-reflex pathway. It is generally free of side effects; however, its effectiveness in suppressing cough is variable and unpredictable. Case series have reported benefit from off-label use of gabapentin or amitriptyline

off-label /ˈɒfˌleɪbl/ adj. 超说明书用药的，未经临床试验认可的

for chronic idiopathic cough. Novel cough suppressants without the limitations of currently available agents are greatly needed. Approaches that are being explored include the development of neurokinin receptor antagonists, type 1 vanilloid receptor antagonists, and

vanilloid /vəˈnɪlɔɪd/ n. 香草酸

novel opioid and opioid-like receptor agonists.

Task 1 Find out the answers to the following questions and then compare your answers with a partner.

1. What could happen when the cough reflex is ineffective?

2. What have been developed to improve cough strength?

3. What is useful in deciding the etiology of a symptomatic cough?

4. When is it appropriate to start cough suppression?

5. Why are novel therapies needed despite the availability of narcotic cough suppressants?

Part II Listening

Task 2 You will hear 20 words or phrases which will be read three times. Write them down on the blanks and check with your partner after you finish.

1. _____   2. _____   3. _____   4. _____

5. _____   6. _____   7. _____   8. _____

9. _____   10. _____   11. _____   12. _____

13. _____   14. _____   15. _____   16. _____

17. _____   18. _____   19. _____   20. _____

Task 3 You are going to hear a passage which will be read three times. Take some notes while you are listening to the passage and then answer the following questions.

1. What is Dr. Fuchs' definition of internal medicine?

_____

2. What conditions may internists handle?

_____

3. Which skills are important for good internists?

_____

Task 4 Read the following passage and make an oral presentation.

When to See an Endocrinologist for Diabetes

If you have been diagnosed with diabetes and you are on insulin or need more specific care, you may be sent to a diabetes specialist by your primary care provider. This specialist is called an endocrinologist, specializing in disorders of the endocrine system. This system produces hormones that regulate metabolism, reproduction, and homeostasis.

What Is an Endocrinologist?

An endocrinologist may provide care in a specialized endocrinology practice, such as one that focuses on diabetes and endocrinology, or split their time by seeing both endocrinology and general internal medicine patients.

Endocrinologists treat diabetes, a disease of the pancreas, and diseases that affect other endocrine systems such as the thyroid, pituitary gland, and adrenal glands. These diseases may include but are not limited to: Hyperthyroidism and hypothyroidism; Pituitary diseases such as pituitary tumors or producing too much or too little pituitary hormones; Sex hormone abnormalities; Reproductive disorders; Osteoporosis; Lipid metabolism.

When to See an Endocrinologist for Diabetes

While you may be diagnosed with type 1 or type 2 diabetes by your primary care provider, sometimes you may need to see an endocrinologist to help you manage your diabetes. This depends on your diabetes type and your individual situation.

In certain cases, such as if you have uncomplicated type 2 diabetes, you may never need to see a diabetes healthcare provider because you can manage the disease through lifestyle changes with your primary provider's guidance. In other more complicated cases, such as with type 1 diabetes, your primary healthcare provider will recommend seeing an endocrinologist.

Though your primary healthcare provider can help guide you as to whether you need to see an endocrinologist for diabetes, there are other reasons why you might choose to or need to see an endocrinologist:

1. Communication: If you feel like your healthcare provider is not listening to your concerns or understanding them, you might see a specialist who can focus on care for your diabetes.

2. Education: While primary healthcare providers are very knowledgeable, you might still have trouble finding specific information relating to diabetes. In this case, an endocrinologist can help you form a diabetes care team to receive diabetes education.

3. Complications: If you are experiencing complications with your diabetes, such as open sores on your feet or problems with your eyes, kidneys, or nerves, a specialist can help manage these symptoms and prevent further damage.

4. Conventional treatments don't work: Your primary care provider may be doing the best they can with the knowledge they have, but if your treatments aren't working, it may be time to see a specialist.

5. Complex treatments: If you take three or more injections a day or use an insulin pump, an endocrinologist can ensure you receive the best recommendations for managing treatment.

Whether or not you see an endocrinologist, remember that you are the most important person on your diabetes care team. You know your body and symptoms better than anyone else.

When it comes to making the choices that impact your treatment plan—when and how you take insulin or medications, what food you eat, the exercise you do—you are in charge.

What to Expect

To help you best manage your diabetes, an endocrinologist will help you by making sure you understand the disease process first. They will then discuss treatment options and how best to manage the disease.

1. Initial exam: In your initial exam, your endocrinologist may go over lab results and discuss your diagnosis. They may then prescribe medications and make sure that you are educated on how to administer these drugs properly, especially if you are prescribed insulin. Your healthcare provider may also discuss lifestyle modifications such as a nutritional and exercise plan that can help you manage your diabetes. Your practitioner will go over any complications that could arise with diabetes and make sure you understand what is to be expected and when to seek additional medical help. Your healthcare provider may also talk to you about how living with diabetes can affect your mental health as well. They will also make sure that your overall health is being taken care of too.

2. Regular visits: During regular visits with your endocrinologist, your healthcare provider will go over your current treatment plan, ask if you have any new symptoms or concerns, and check to ensure that you are doing OK in managing your diabetes. Sometimes, you can feel overwhelmed at a healthcare provider's appointment and forget your concerns. You may consider writing down your questions before seeing your practitioner so that you can make sure that everything is addressed. You should plan to see your healthcare provider at least twice a year, but more often if you are having difficulty managing your diabetes or reaching your blood glucose, blood pressure, or cholesterol goals. Depending on the information you provide at your regular visits and any test results they receive, they may change your treatment plan.

Managing Diabetes

While it may take time to adjust to life with diabetes, creating a self-care plan with the guidance of your healthcare provider can help you manage diabetes in long term. By taking care of yourself every day, you can live a long, healthy life with diabetes.

A typical management plan includes regular visits with your

healthcare provider to check blood glucose levels and other markers of health such as blood pressure and cholesterol levels. Your practitioner or care team may also help you create a nutritional plan that helps you regulate blood glucose, blood pressure, and cholesterol.

Making sure to get regular exercise is also important to managing diabetes as is taking all medications as prescribed, even if you start to feel better. Depending on your type of diabetes, you may also need to check your blood glucose levels on a regular basis, not just at healthcare provider's appointments.

Creating a diabetes team: To help you manage every aspect of your health and diabetes, you may find that creating a team of different healthcare providers can be incredibly resourceful. These health providers can include: Primary care provider—A healthcare provider who can oversee your entire health and well-being along with your diabetes; Endocrinologist—A healthcare provider who will provide specialized diabetic care; Ophthalmologist/optometrist—A healthcare provider who can diagnose and treat eye disorders; Podiatrist—A healthcare provider who can treat feet and lower leg problems such as nerve damage and ulcers; Pharmacist—A professional who can advise you on your medications and how to take them properly; Dentist—A healthcare provider who can monitor your oral health, which impacts your overall health; Registered nurse/nurse navigator—Nurses who can help coordinate your medical care; Registered dietitian—A healthcare professional who can help you figure out what to eat and drink to manage your diabetes; Certified diabetes care and education specialist (CDCES)—Professionals who can help you manage the things you need to do to take care of your diabetes; Mental health professional—Healthcare providers and therapists who can help you deal with the challenges of day-to-day life with diabetes and any emotions that come along with this; Fitness professional—A physical therapist, physiologist, or personal trainer who can help you stay active.

Task 5 **Theme-related discussion.**

Internal medicine deals with the diagnosis and treatment of diseases affecting the internal organs of the body, especially in adults. Ancient Greek physicians studied and gave the name "diabetes" to a chronic disease characterized by excessive urination. The prevalence of diabetes has been gradually increasing worldwide. Many diabetes patients come to the Department of Internal Medicine for help.

Please watch the MOOC, think about it, and discuss the following questions with your partner.

1. What are the complications of diabetes?

2. What are the measures for diabetes patients to lead a healthy life?

Part Ⅳ   Word Formation

chemical compound [英] 化合物

  -in/-ine [拉] 化合物

    angiotensin /ˌændʒɪəˈtensɪn/ *n*. 血管紧张素

    amitriptyline /ˌæmɪˈtrɪptiliːn/ *n*. 阿米替林

    codeine /ˈkəʊdiːn/ *n*. 可待因，甲基吗啡

windpipe [英] 气管

  trache(o)- [希] 气管

    tracheostomy /ˌtreɪkɪˈɒstəmi/ *n*. 气管切开术

    tracheobronchitis /ˌtreɪkiəbrɒŋˈkaɪtɪs/ *n*. 气管支气管炎

    tracheal /trəˈkiːəl/ *adj*. 气管的

resemblance to [英] 类……的，似……的

  -oid [希] 类……的，似……的

    mucoid /ˈmjuːkɒɪd/ *adj*. 黏液状的

    steroid /ˈsterɒɪd/ *n*. 类固醇

    carotenoid /kəˈrɒtənɒɪd/ *n*. 类胡萝卜素

new [英] 新的

  neo- [拉] 新的

    neoplastic /ˌniːəʊˈplæstɪk/ *adj*. 赘生的，肿瘤的

    neonatal /ˌniːəʊˈneɪtəl/ *adj*. 新生儿的

    neocortex /ˌniːəʊˈkɔːteks/ *n*. （大脑）新皮质

eating, ingestion [英] 吃，吞食

  phag(o)- [希] 吃，吞食

    macrophage /ˈmækrəfeɪdʒ/ *n*. 巨噬细胞

esophageal /iːˌsɒfəˈdʒiːəl/ *adj.* 食管的

phagolysosome /ˌfæɡəʊˈlaɪsəsəʊm/ *n.* 吞噬溶酶体

Task 6 **Match each of the following terms with its definition.**

1	neogenetic	A	hemorrhage from the mucous membrane of the trachea
2	phagocytable	B	a hormone that helps regulate blood pressure
3	angiotensin	C	inspection of the interior of the trachea and bronchi
4	fibroid	D	susceptible to cell eating
5	tracheorrhagia	E	composed of or resembling fibrous tissue
6	tracheobronchoscopy	F	of or characterized by the process of regeneration or of producing a new formation

Task 7 **Fill in the blanks with words or phrases given in the box. Change the form where necessary.**

macrophage	neoplasm	tracheobronchial	insulin
phagophobia	tracheostomy	steroid	neonate
epinephrine	lipoid		

1. _____ pneumonia has long been described as aspiration of oil into the lungs and has been associated with e-cigarette use in some case reports.

2. A tumor, also known as a _____, is an abnormal lump or growth that forms in or on the body.

3. We describe a case of _____ in a 15-year-old girl who was treated successfully with low-dose aripiprazole as an augmentation therapy after she witnessed her father choking while eating chicken.

4. The trachea, bronchi and bronchioles form the _____ tree—a system of airways that allow passage of air into the lungs, where gas exchange occurs.

5. _____ are cells of the innate immune system and represent an important component of the first-line defense against pathogens and tumor cells.

6. If _____ are taken daily, for long periods of time, they can cause adrenal gland suppression.

7. _____ injection is a medicine that treats severe allergic reactions and low blood pressure.

8. This chapter provides guidance on essential newborn care and the management of problems in _____ and young infants, from birth to 2 months of age.

9. Hypoglycemia is the most common and severe side effect of _____ , occurring in approximately 16% of type I and 10% of type II diabetic patients.

10. Percutaneous _____ is a minimally invasive procedure doctors perform to establish an artificial airway.

Part V Fast Reading

Helicobacter Pylori

Helicobacter pylori unusual name identifies specific bacteria that can cause infection of the stomach. This infection can contribute to the development of diseases, such as dyspepsia (heartburn, bloating and nausea), gastritis (inflammation of the stomach), and ulcers in the stomach and duodenum. It will be useful to know some things about the upper digestive tract to understand how and where Helicobacter pylori infection can occur.

When food is swallowed, it passes through the esophagus (the tube that connects the throat to the stomach). It then enters the larger upper part of the stomach. A strong acid that helps to break down the food is secreted in the stomach. The narrower, lower part of the stomach is called the antrum. The antrum contracts frequently and vigorously, grinding up the food and squirting it into the small intestine. The duodenum is the first part of the small intestine, just beyond the stomach. The stomach, including the antrum, is covered by a layer of mucus that protects it from the strong stomach acid.

It is known that alcohol, aspirin, and arthritis drugs such as ibuprofen can disrupt the protective mucous layer. This allows the strong stomach acid to injure underlying stomach cells. In some people, corticosteroids, smoking, and stress appear to contribute in some way. Until the mid 1980s, it was felt that one or more of these factors working together led to the development of gastritis and ulcers. Since that time, evidence has been mounting that *Helicobacter pylori* (*H. pylori*) has a major role in causing these diseases.

The Infection

H. *pylori* is a fragile bacteria that has found an ideal home in the protective mucous layer of the stomach. These bacteria have long threads protruding from them that attach to the underlying stomach cells. The mucous layer that protects the stomach cells from acid also protects H. *pylori*. These bacteria do not actually invade the stomach cells as certain other bacteria can. The infection, however, is very real and it does cause the body to react. Infection-fighting white blood cells move into the area, and the body even develops H. *pylori* antibodies in the blood.

H. *pylori* infection probably occurs when an individual swallows the bacteria in food, fluid, or perhaps from contaminated utensils. The infection is likely one of the most common worldwide. The rate of infection increases with age, so it occurs more often in older people. It also occurs frequently in young people in the developing countries of the world, since the infection tends to be more common where sanitation is poor or living quarters are cramped. In many cases it does not produce symptoms. In other words, the infection can occur without the person knowing it. The infection remains localized to the gastric area, and probably persists unless specific treatment is given.

How is H. *pylori* Infection Diagnosed?

There are currently three ways to diagnose H. *pylori* infection. During endoscopy (a visual exam of the stomach through a thin, lighted, flexible tube), the physician can remove small bits of tissue through the tube. The tissue is then tested for the bacteria. A breath test is now available. In this test, a substance called urea is given by mouth. A strong enzyme in the bacteria breaks down the urea into carbon dioxide, which is then exhaled and can be measured. And finally, there is a blood test that measures the protein antibodies against these bacteria that are present in the blood. This antibody can mean the infection is present, or that it was present in the past and is now cleared. In other words, a person can have a positive blood test but no infection.

Gastritis and Dyspepsia

The symptoms are discomfort, bloating, nausea and perhaps vomiting. The person may also have symptoms that suggest ulcers—burning or pain in the upper abdomen, usually occurring about an hour or so after meals or even during the night. The symptoms are often relieved temporarily by antacids, milk, or medications that reduce stomach acidity. Yet, the physician does not find an ulcer when the patient is tested by X-ray or endoscopy. When *H. pylori* is found in the stomach, it is tempting to believe that it is the cause of the symptoms, although this connection is not yet clear cut. The physician will usually prescribe antibiotic therapy to see if clearing the infection relieves symptoms.

Ulcers

Stomach Ulcers: With stomach ulcers, *H. pylori* infection is found in 60 to 80 percent of the cases. Again, it is still uncertain how the infection acts to cause the ulcer. It probably weakens the protective mucous layer of the stomach. This allows acid to seep in and injure the underlying stomach cells. However, there is still a great deal of research to be done to unravel this relationship.

Duodenal ulcers: In times past, physicians were taught "no acid, no ulcer." The medical profession felt the single most important factor causing duodenal ulcers to form was strong stomach acid. Research has now shown that over 90% of all patients who develop duodenal ulcers have *H. pylori* infection in the stomach as well. Medical studies are under way to determine the relationship between the two and how an infection in the stomach can be related to a duodenal ulcer. Acid is still important; patients without acid in the stomach never get duodenal ulcers. However, physicians now accept the fact that the infection is directly related to the development of duodenal ulcers. It is now rather easy to clear duodenal ulcers with the strong acid-reducing medicines available. But, the ulcers will usually recur unless the *H. pylori* infection is also cleared from the stomach.

Stomach Cancer and Lymphoma

These two types of cancer are now known to be related to *H. pylori* bacteria. This does not mean that all people with

H. pylori infection will develop cancer; in fact, very few do. However, it is likely that if the infection is present for a long time, perhaps from childhood, these cancers may then develop.

When is Treatment Necessary?

Since the infection is so common, it is sometimes recommended that no treatment be given when there are no symptoms. However, these recommendations may change as more research develops. Increasingly, physicians are treating the acute ulcer with acid-reducing medicines and treating the infection with antibiotics. Interestingly, one of these antibiotics is a bismuth compound that is available over-the-counter as Pepto-Bismol. It is also available as a generic drug called bismuth subsalicylate. The bismuth part of the medicine actually kills the bacteria. However, do not go to the drugstore and purchase a bottle of Pepto-Bismol, expecting this alone to cure the infection. *H. pylori* is buried deep in the stomach mucus, so it is difficult to get rid of this infection. Several antibiotic drugs are always used together to prevent the bacteria from developing resistance to any one of them. Current medical studies are being done to develop easier treatment programs for this difficult infection.

Summary

H. pylori is a very common infection of the stomach. It may be the most common infection in the world. It is now clear that the infection is directly related to the development of stomach and duodenal ulcers, and it is likely that it may be related to cancers involving the stomach. There are several diagnostic tests available, and effective treatment can prevent the recurrence of ulcers and perhaps the development of cancer.

Task 8 **Read the passage and decide whether the statements are true or false. If it is true, write "T". If it is not, write "F".**

1. The infection of *Helicobacter pylori* can contribute to the development of diseases, such as dyspepsia, gastritis, and ulcers in the stomach and duodenum. (　　)

2. Strong stomach acid is the single most important factor causing duodenal ulcers.

(　　)

3. The infection rate of *H. pylori* decreases with age. ( )

4. Breath test, blood test and endoscopy are the three ways to diagnose *H. pylori* infection. ( )

5. Doctors may prescribe several antibiotics together for the treatment of *H. pylori* infection. ( )

Task 9 **Read the passage again and write a two-hundred-word synopsis.**

Part VI Translation

Task 10 **Analyze the following sentences and then put them into Chinese.**

1. At the other extreme, excessive coughing can be exhausting; can be complicated by emesis, syncope, muscular pain, or rib fractures; and can aggravate abdominal or inguinal hernias and urinary incontinence.

_____

_____

2. During regular visits with your endocrinologist, your healthcare provider will go over your current treatment plan, ask if you have any new symptoms or concerns, and check to ensure that you are doing OK in managing your diabetes.

_____

_____

3. It will be useful to know some things about the upper digestive tract to understand how and where *Helicobacter pylori* infection can occur.

_____

_____

医学翻译技巧

并列句中的省略

并列句中的省略是指翻译或写作并列句时省略后一个句子中与前一个句子相同的部分。

例1 尽管接种了疫苗,仍发生了一例肺炎双球菌脑膜炎、一例肺炎双球菌菌血症。

Despite vaccination, one patient developed pneumococcal meningitis and another, pneumococcal bacteremia.

两句都使用了S(主语)+V(谓语)+O(宾语)结构,主语都是病人,而且后一个句子里的谓语动词与前一个句子的谓语动词都是实义动词,且时态相同,所以翻译时省略谓语动词 developed,并用逗号做了提示。

例2 在一个九口之家,有2人患系统性红斑狼疮,另7人梅毒血清学检验为阳性。

In a family of 9 members, 2 had systemic lupus erythematosus and 7 (had) positive serological test results for syphilis.

本句两个并列句结构相同,两个动词的功能作用和句子采用的时态相同,所以省略后一个句子的动词 had,可不用逗号提示。

例3 作者综述了该综合征,并报导一例患者的麻醉方法。

The syndrome is reviewed and the anesthetic management of a case (is) described.

本句的两个并列句的结构都是:主语 + 被动语态,后一句与前一句的助动词相同,时态也相同,所以省略后一个助动词 is,可不用逗号提示。

但是,下面的句子翻译时不可作省略处理:

例4 作者发现黏膜浅层病变的发病率高,并强调了这些病变早期诊断的重要性。

A high incidence of superficial mucosal lesions was found, and the importance of early investigation in the diagnosis of these lesions is stressed.

本句中两个并列句的动词都是助动词 be,但它们的时态不同,所以后一个句子中的助动词 be 不可省略。

例5 在这些患者中,全血细胞扫描异常者12例(36%),其中11例与临床相符。

The whole blood cell scan was abnormal in 12 (36%) of these, and a good clinical correlation was obtained in 11 of the 12.

本句中两个并列句的动词都是 was,但前一个 was 是系动词,后一个 was 是助动词,所以后一个句子中的 was 不可省略。

Task 11 Translate the following sentences into English.

1. 病例组使用手提电话的平均时间是 2.8 年,而对照组使用手提电话的平均时间是 2.7 年。

_____

2. 病人经过 3 至 5 年的随访,良好 6 例,进步 4 例,有效率达 88.9%。

_____

3. 在这些病人中，16 例接受了手术治疗，8 例接受了保守治疗。

_____

4. 应尽快切开病人的气管，立即取出异物。

_____

5. 有些病只在人与人之间传播，而有些病仅在动物之间传播。

_____

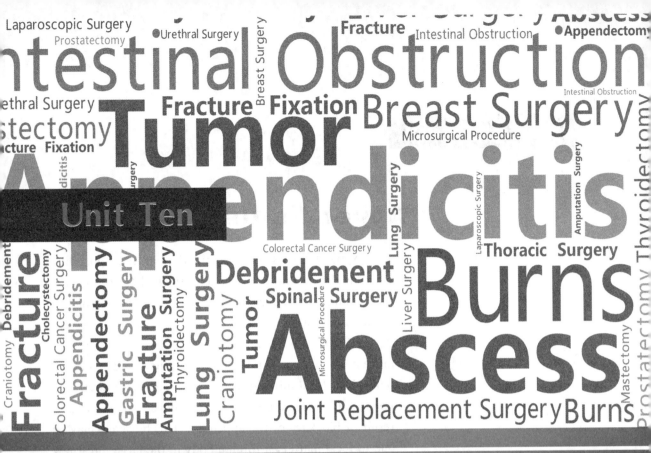

Unit Ten

Surgery

✓课文音频
✓听力音频
✓在线课程
✓课件申请

Appendicitis

Appendicitis is an inflammation of the appendix, which is the worm-shaped pouch attached to the cecum, the beginning of the large intestine. The appendix has no known function in the body, but it can become diseased. Appendicitis is a medical emergency, and if it is left untreated, the appendix may **rupture** and cause a potentially fatal infection. The causes of appendicitis are not totally understood, but are believed to occur as a result of blockage of the appendix. This blockage may be due to fecal matter, a foreign body in the large intestine, cancerous tumors, a **parasite infestation**, or swelling from an infection.

The distinguishing symptom of appendicitis is the migration of pain to the lower right corner of the abdomen. The abdomen often becomes rigid and tender to the touch. The patient may bend the knees in reaction to the pain. Increased rigidity and tenderness indicate an increased likelihood of **perforation** and **peritonitis**. Loss of appetite is very common, accompanied by a low-grade fever, and occasionally there is **constipation** or diarrhea, as well as nausea. Unfortunately, these signs and symptoms may vary widely. Atypical symptoms are particularly present in pregnant women, the elderly, and young children.

A careful examination is the best way to diagnose appendicitis. It is often difficult even for experienced physicians to distinguish the symptoms of appendicitis from those of other abdominal disorders. The physician will ask questions regarding the nature and history of the pain, as well doing an abdominal exam to feel for inflammation, tenderness, and rigidity. Bowel sounds

rupture /ˈrʌptʃə/ n.& v. 破裂

parasite /ˈpærəsaɪt/ n. 寄生虫
infestation /ˌɪnfeˈsteɪʃn/ n. 侵染

perforation /pɜːfəˈreɪʃ(ə)n/ n. 穿孔
peritonitis /ˌperɪtəʊˈnaɪtɪs/ n. 腹膜炎

constipation /ˌkɒnstɪˈpeɪʃən/ n. 便秘

will be decreased or absent. A blood test will be given, because an increased white cell count may help confirm a diagnosis of appendicitis. Urinalysis may help to rule out a urinary tract infection that can mimic appendicitis. In cases with a questionable diagnosis, other tests, such as a computed tomography scan (CT) or ultrasound may be performed to help with diagnosis without resorting to surgery. Abdominal X rays, however, are not of much value except when the appendix has ruptured.

urinalysis /ˌjuːrɪ'nælɪsɪs/ n. 尿液分析

The treatment for sudden, severe appendicitis is surgery to remove the appendix, called an appendectomy. An appendectomy may be done by opening the abdomen in the standard operating technique, or through laparoscopy, in which a small incision is made through the navel. Recovery may be faster with a laparoscopy than with an ordinary appendectomy. An appendectomy should be performed within 48 hours of the first appearance of symptoms, to avoid a rupture of the appendix and peritonitis. Antibiotics are given before surgery in case peritonitis has already taken hold. If peritonitis is discovered, the abdomen must also be irrigated and drained of pus, and then treated with multiple antibiotics for 7—14 days. Appendicitis is usually treated successfully by appendectomy. Unless there are complications, the patient should recover without further problems. The mortality rate in cases without complications is less than 0.1%. When an appendix has ruptured, or a severe infection has developed, the likelihood is higher for complications, with slower recovery, or death from disease. There are higher rates of perforation and mortality among children and the elderly.

appendectomy /ˌæpən'dektəmi/ n. 阑尾切除术

laparoscopy /ˌlæpə'rɒskəpi/ n. 腹腔镜检查
incision /ɪn'sɪʒən/ n. 切口
navel /'neɪvəl/ n. 脐

irrigate /'ɪrɪgeɪt/ vt. 冲洗
pus /pʌs/ n. 脓

complication /ˌkɒmplɪ'keɪʃən/ n. 并发症

mortality /mɔː'tælɪti/ n. 死亡率

Task 1 Find out the answers to the following questions and then compare your answers with a partner.

1. Is it true that the causes of appendicitis are known to us?

2. What is the distinguishing symptom of appendicitis?

3. Are abdominal X rays of any value when the appendix has ruptured?

4. May the recovery be faster with a laparoscopy than with an ordinary appendectomy?

5. When should an appendectomy be performed? Why?

Part Ⅱ Listening

Task 2 You will hear 20 words or phrases which will be read three times. Write them down on the blanks and check with your partner after you finish.

1. _____ 2. _____ 3. _____ 4. _____

5. _____ 6. _____ 7. _____ 8. _____

9. _____ 10. _____ 11. _____ 12. _____

13. _____ 14. _____ 15. _____ 16. _____

17. _____ 18. _____ 19. _____ 20. _____

Task 3 You are going to hear a passage which will be read three times. Take some notes while you are listening to the passage and then answer the following questions.

1. What may surgeons do in their daily work?

_____

2. In addition to superior academic ability, what other skills may surgeons need to have?

_____

3. Why is it important for surgeons to learn new technologies and continually develop their skills?

_____

Task 4 Read the following passage and make an oral presentation.

Artificial Intelligence Expedites Brain Tumor Diagnosis during Surgery

For patients with a brain tumor, the first step in treatment is often surgery to remove as much of the mass as possible. A tumor sample obtained and analyzed during surgery can help to precisely diagnose the tumor and define the margins between tumor and healthy brain tissue.

However, such intraoperative pathology analysis takes time—the sample must be processed, stained, and analyzed by a pathologist while the surgeon and patient wait for the results. Now, a new study shows that a process combining an advanced imaging technology and artificial intelligence (AI) can accurately diagnose brain tumors in fewer than 3 minutes during surgery. The approach was also able to accurately distinguish tumor tissue from healthy tissue.

"This technology is especially encouraging for patients with newly detected tumors and patients with recurrent tumors who are undergoing second or third surgeries," said Daniel Orringer, M.D., of NYU Langone Health, who helped lead the study.

This study, the research team wrote, opens the door to "providing unparalleled access to intraoperative tissue diagnosis at the bedside during surgery" while "reducing the risk of removing ... normal tissue adjacent to a tumor."

Kareem Zaghloul, M.D., Ph.D., a neurosurgeon in NIH's Surgical Neurology Branch who was not involved in the research, said he is encouraged by the study's results. "This technology could help inform how aggressive or conservative surgery needs to be," Dr. Zaghloul said.

Applying Imaging and AI Technology

In the study, a research team led by Dr. Orringer and Todd Hollon, M. D., chief neurosurgery resident at the University of Michigan, wanted to test whether they could combine an imaging technology called stimulated Raman histology (SRH) with the predictive power of AI to improve current intraoperative pathology practice.

SRH, a specialized form of microscopy, can be used to visualize fresh tissue samples directly in the operating room, even producing the same sort of "staining" that pathologists apply to frozen tissue samples to analyze cellular structure. At the University of Michigan, surgical teams are already using an SRH system for some brain tumor and head and neck cancer procedures.

AI involves using powerful computers to perform tasks that are typically associated with human intelligence. A type of AI known as deep learning uses complex mathematical algorithms, sometimes called convolutional neural networks, to extract features from data that it is then "trained" on.

This training allows the algorithm to recognize patterns and perform tasks such as analyzing images. In medicine, for example, such algorithms are being studied to see if they can help assess mammograms, detect precancerous tissue in the cervix, or detect cancerous moles more accurately.

To combine the power of the SRH imager with AI, the researchers began by training an algorithm on SRH-produced images of brain tumor tissue. For the training, they used more than 2.5 million tumor tissue images from 415 patients. The images covered three nontumor-tissue classifications, including healthy grey or white matter, and the 10 most common brain tumor types, which account for more than 90% of all brain tumor diagnoses in the United States.

"A major initial challenge was determining the ideal size and resolution of images to train the algorithm," Dr. Hollon said. Once these ideal parameters were determined, the algorithm learned to classify tissue samples as definitive tumor, nontumor tissue, or nondiagnostic (meaning they couldn't be analyzed by AI).

Testing in a Clinical Trial

To explore the clinical value of the SRH-AI technology for diagnosing brain tumors, the researchers enrolled nearly 280 patients in a clinical trial, all of whom agreed to allow surgeons to collect additional tumor tissue beyond what would usually be collected but in a way that would not pose additional risks.

Tissue specimens were divided into two and analyzed using the new technology (SRH images classified by the algorithm) in the operating room and conventional laboratory pathology (tissues processed, stained, and analyzed by a pathologist) to see if the new technology was as accurate as the conventional technology.

That proved to be the case. The algorithm correctly diagnosed brain tumors 94.6% of the time, while conventional pathologist-based analysis had an overall accuracy rate of 93.9%.

In the instances where tissue specimens were incorrectly classified by the algorithm, a pathologist had made the correct diagnosis. And in the instances where pathologists incorrectly classified a sample, the algorithm had made the correct diagnosis.

The researchers noted that the ability of the AI technology and pathologists to cross-check each other highlights the need for pathologists to work alongside the AI technology to interpret challenging cases and ensure the highest diagnostic accuracy possible.

Improving Surgical Accuracy

The extent of tumor removal can be determined during surgery as well as with a post-operative MRI scan that shows how complete the removal was. While removing as much tumor as possible during surgery can improve how long patients live, removing too much healthy brain tissue during surgery can have serious and harmful consequences for a patient, such as impaired motor function, memory loss, or vision problems.

To address this, the researchers also looked at the ability of the new technology to distinguish tumor tissue from healthy brain tissue while the patient is still in surgery.

Because tumor cells can sometimes infiltrate healthy tissues, it can be difficult to identify the border between tumor and healthy tissue with the naked eye during surgery. By breaking up each specimen image into smaller "patches," the AI technology allows surgeons to quickly and clearly identify areas containing tumor or healthy tissue.

Using SRH-AI technology, Dr. Orringer said, "we can ... visualize tumor cells that would otherwise be invisible during surgery."

And since "a patient's prognosis is dependent on the extent of resection," said Dr. Zaghloul, having better information on the brain-tumor margin "could result in better treatment outcomes for patients and fewer surgery-related complications due to healthy tissue being preserved."

The Future of AI in Brain Tumors

Before the new technology can be expanded to other centers and institutions, "robust testing with more patients and expanding the technology to include rare brain tumors are greatly needed," Dr. Zaghloul said.

The SRH imager is being used at several major cancer centers across the United States today. Both AI and SRH imaging are emerging technologies, so there will be challenges to integrating them into care, Dr. Orringer explained, such as financial or regulatory issues as well as clinician training.

Even so, Dr. Orringer is hopeful that use of the SRH-AI technology will expand in the future, including at centers with limited pathology resources and for potential use in a number of different cancer types.

Task 5 **Theme-related discussion.**

Artificial intelligence (AI) achievements have transformed modern surgery toward more precise and autonomous interventions for treating acute and chronic symptoms. A new study shows that a process combining advanced imaging technology and artificial intelligence can accurately diagnose brain tumors in fewer than 3 minutes during surgery.

Please watch the MOOC, think about it, and discuss the following questions with your partner.

1. What are the advantages and challenges of using AI in surgery?

2. What are the new requirements for surgeons in the face of the application of AI in surgery?

Part IV Word Formation

urine [英] 尿

  urin(o)- [拉] 尿

    urinogenital /ˌjuːrɪnəʊˈdʒenɪtəl/ adj. 泌尿生殖的

    urinaserum /ˌjuːrɪˈnæsərəm/ n. 尿(蛋白)免疫血清

    uriniferous /ˌjuːrɪˈnɪfərəs/ adj. 输尿的

  -uria [希] 尿(症)

    glycosuria /ˌglaɪkəʊˈsjuːrɪə/ n. 糖尿

    hematuria /ˌhiːməˈtjuːrɪə/ n. 血尿, 尿血

    polyuria /ˌpɒliˈjuːrɪə/ n. 多尿

around [英] 周围, 环绕

  peri- [希] 周, 周围

    peripheral /pəˈrɪfərəl/ adj. 外周的

    periarthritis /ˌperɪɑːˈθraɪtɪs/ n. 关节周炎

    pericardial /ˌperɪˈkɑːdɪəl/ adj. 心包的

spectacles [英] 镜

  -scope, -scopy [希] 镜; 镜检

    endoscopy /enˈdɒskəpi/ n. 内镜检查术

    hysteroscope /ˈhɪstərəskəʊp/ n. 宫腔镜

    laparoscopy /ˌlæpəˈrɒskəpi/ n. 腹腔镜检查

stone [英] 石头

  -lith [希] 石, 结石

    broncholith /ˈbrɒŋkəlɪθ/ n. 支气管石

    cholelith /ˈkəʊlilɪθ/ n. 胆石

    urolith /ˈjuːrəlɪθ/ n. 尿石

twelve [英] 十二

  duoden(o)- [拉] 十二

    duodenoscope /ˌdjuːəʊˈdiːnəskəʊp/ n. 十二指肠镜

    duodenum /ˌdjuːəˈdiːnəm/ n. 十二指肠

    duodenectomy /ˌdjuːədəˈnektəmi/ n. 十二指肠切除术

ball-like germ [英] 球菌

  -coccus [拉] 球菌 -cocci (pl.) 球菌

    staphylococcus /ˌstæfɪləʊˈkɒkəs/ n. 葡萄球菌

streptococci /ˌstreptəʊˈkɒksaɪ/ *n*. 链球菌

shape［英］成形

-plasty［希］成形术，整形术

osteoplasty /ˈɒstiəˌplæsti/ *n*. 骨整形术，骨成形术

gastroplasty /ˈgæstrəʊˌplæsti/ *n*. 胃成形术

enteroplasty /ˈentərəʊˌplæsti/ *n*. 肠成形术

Task 6 **Match each of the following terms with its definition.**

1 endoscopy   A spherical Gram-positive parasitic bacteria

2 urinometer   B the dense, fibrous, connective layer of tissue covering all
                         bones

3 staphylococcus   C a device for determining the specific gravity of urine

4 hematuria   D visual examination of the internal organs

5 nephrolithotomy   E the presence of blood in the urine

6 periosteum   F a procedure used to remove kidney stones from the body

Task 7 **Fill in the blanks with words or phrases given in the box. Change the form where necessary.**

polyuria	urinalysis	pericardium	laparoscope
urinate	peritoneal	streptococci	cholelith
duodenum	aortoplasty		

1. Cases that had _____ only in the gallbladder were excluded from the study.

2. Laparoscopy is a type of surgery that gets its name from the _____, a slender tool that has a tiny video camera and light on the end.

3. In this retrospective analysis that includes 253 patients with nonreinforced reduction ascending _____ due to ascending aortic aneurysms, the safety and efficacy of this strategy were confirmed.

4. A test called a _____ checks a sample of your urine to see if there's blood in it.

5. Viridans _____ inhabit the mouth of healthy people but can invade the bloodstream, especially in people with periodontal inflammation, and infect heart valves.

6. Alcohol and caffeine can irritate the bladder and increase the urge to _____.

7. Pericarditis is inflammation of the _____, a sac-like structure with two thin layers of tissue that surround the heart to hold it in place and help it work.

8. The stomach is a hollow intraperitoneal organ in the left upper quadrant of the abdomen, between the esophagus and the _____ in the gastrointestinal tract.

9. Solute-induced _____ can be seen in hospitalized patients after a high solute load from exogenous protein administration or following relief of urinary obstruction.

10. _____ dialysis is a treatment for kidney failure that uses the lining of your abdomen, or belly, to filter your blood inside your body.

Part V   Fast Reading

Traveling Nurse

A good nurse would not pursue becoming a traveling nurse simply because of the potential earnings involved. A good nurse would not pursue the career in order to have shorter shifts and spend more time with their family. Good nurses don't become nurses because they are looking for careers that require a less amount of physical exertion. A good nurse does not become a nurse because they cannot be bothered to study to become a doctor. Nurses become nurses because they feel a greater need to assist in the treatment and rehabilitation of sick or injured persons.

There are several steps involved before one can become a traveling nurse. The first step is to become enrolled in an approved nursing qualification program. There is currently a shortage of educational nursing programs in the US, so it is advised to enroll as early as possible as places may fill quickly. Once the nursing student has been accepted into an educational nursing institution the student can then choose to pursue a variety of degrees including an associate degree, a bachelor's degree, a master's degree, or even a nursing doctorate.

It is a requirement for traveling nurses to be RN-registered nurses, so they can perform all the required tasks by law—such as diagnosing conditions and administering treatments. It is also advised for traveling nurses to have at least 1-year experience before embarking on their traveling nurse journey. This will place them in the best position to attract the best work on their trip.

Office nurses essentially are located in the doctor's office. Most office nurses are responsible for administering medications to patients, preparing the patient for their examination, and helping to dress wounds. Office nurses have a fairly regular schedule, and more often than not are full-time so there are fewer opportunities for traveling nurses—except in situations such as maternity leave.

Another form of nurse is a home nurse. A home nurse is a nurse who travels to the patients home to treat them there—often because they are less mobile or elderly. In extreme cases a home nurse will be required to move into the patients' home to treat them on a more regular basis. Some home nurses work as midwives to help them deliver the child from their home. There are certainly opportunities for traveling nurses in home nursing. Quite often the assignments are shorter, and obviously less formal due to the nature of working from someone's home. Home nursing is a good option for a lot of traveling nurses.

Hospital nurses are essentially nurses that work in hospitals. The majority of work for traveling nurses will be located in hospitals—and will be widely available throughout the world. A traveling nurse always has a length of assignment of placement in a hospital, this means they know how long they are going to be there and can plan how to make the most of their time. This often results in a greater interest in their work than is displayed by regular full time nurses.

A good traveling nurse requires flexibility. This is perhaps the most crucial aspect of becoming a traveling nurse. As one may be traveling from place to place at the mercy of the traveling nurse agency, it is important to be flexible. Obviously it is completely fine to inform your agency which shifts you wish to take, and the locations you would prefer to work in—however flexibility will always be rewarded.

It is not vital, but being a more outgoing and communicative person will benefit your career as a traveling nurse. As communication between patient and staff is such a large art of what a nurse does on a daily basis, this character trait will be observed and rewarded.

In becoming a good traveling nurse all aspects of nursing need to be first considered. Second to this a greater flexibility and outgoing personality will greatly serve to improve your traveling nurse career. There are many benefits for being a traveling nurse, and good traveling nurses will be duly rewarded with the best work and conditions.

There are some differences in the nursing practice between Britain and the US. A nursing licensed in Britain may practice anywhere in the country and in some foreign countries, but in the United States, the nurse must apply in every state where she hopes to work. In Britain, a nurse is a highly respected, devoted woman, or occasionally man with a vast amount of responsibility. The patients have great belief in her judgment and advice, the doctor relies on her reports and seldom interferes in a nursing duty. What's more, the nurse is always consulted about the patient's requirements and his progress. And the nurse is a member of the health team who sees the patient most frequently. So to the patient, she is the most familiar person in the strange hospital world.

But in the United States, the patient is likely to be under the care of the same doctor in and out of the hospital. So the doctor is the person the patient knows best and the one he trusts most easily. Although the patient's treatment and care are discussed with the nurse, a nurse is not allowed much freedom to advise a patient. But actually, nursing practice is easier in the US. For nurses don't need to write several charges or care for the needs of the patient. Medicines are always kept at hand, and all charges are met by "National Health". And the patients don't have much anxiety and so is more easily cared for while he is in hospital.

Task 8 Read the passage and decide whether the statements are true or false. If it is true, write "T". If it is not, write "F".

1. The first step to be a traveling nurse is to be a doctor. (　)

2. A home nurse can help to deliver a child. (　)

3. The most important quality of being a traveling nurse is to be flexible. (　)

4. A nurse should communicate with the patients and give them advice. (　)

5. There are many nursing programs in US, so one can easily enter a qualified nursing home. (　)

Part Ⅵ Translation

Task 10 Analyze the following sentences and then put them into Chinese.

1. The distinguishing symptom of appendicitis is the migration of pain to the lower right corner of the abdomen. The abdomen often becomes rigid and tender to the touch. The patient may bend the knees in reaction to the pain. Loss of appetite is very common, accompanied by a low-grade fever, and occasionally there is constipation or diarrhea, as well as nausea.

_____

_____

2. A tumor sample obtained and analyzed during surgery can help to precisely diagnose the tumor and define the margins between tumor and healthy brain tissue.

_____

_____

3. Office nurses have a fairly regular schedule, and more often than not are full-time so there are fewer opportunities for traveling nurses—except in situations such as maternity leave.

_____

_____

医学翻译技巧

常用表达

1. 剂量的表示法

剂量的英文单词是 dose 和 dosage。前者表示一次用的剂量,后者表示决定和调整各种剂量的大小、频率与次数。这两个词在英文词典里的含义很清楚,实际应用时却很复杂。

表示一次剂量时只能用 dose,特别要用 a dose of 这个结构:

例 1　用庆大霉素治疗,每次 80 mg,每天 2 次。

　　Therapy with gentamycin in a dose of 80 mg twice daily was instituted.

例2　12名身体健康的人群一次口服100 mg氨酰心安。

A single oral 100 mg <u>dose of</u> atenolol was given to 12 healthy subjects.

表示"一天量"或"总剂量"，dose与dosage可通用。

例3　由于胃肠道不能耐受，故剂量限制在每天50 mg。

Gastrointestinal intolerance restricted <u>dosage/dose</u> to 50 mg daily.

如果泛指剂量，则应用dosage。

例4　在决定剂量方案时，必须知道药物在体内的蓄积程度。

In determining <u>dosage</u> regimens, it is also necessary to know the extent of drug accumulation.

2. 数量增减的表示法

常用的表示数量增加的动词有increase、rise、raise、go up、be up、attain等，表示数量减少的动词有decrease、fall、decline、reduce、drop、lower、go down、be shortened等。另外，介词by可以表示纯增、减数，介词to表示增、减到什么数量。

例5　肺结核的发病率在过去20年里增加将近5倍。

The incidence of the pulmonary tuberculosis <u>has risen by</u> nearly 5 times (five fold) over the last two decades.

例6　总的治疗时间可以减少到15～20天。

The total time of treatment can <u>be reduced to</u> 15—20 days.

3. 极限数的表达

极限数表示某一数量达到多少限度，如高达as high as＋数词，多达as much (many) as＋数词，长达as long as＋数词。

例7　禽流感的潜伏期长达半月之久。

The incubation period of the bird influenza may <u>be as long as</u> half a month.

例8　即使是正常人，左心房压力也有所不同，低可到1毫米汞柱，高可达6毫米汞柱。

The pressure in the left atrium varies, even among normal individuals, from <u>as low as</u> 1 mmHg to <u>as high as</u> 6 mmHg.

4. 一般数值表示法

各类一般数值可用(a＋数值名词＋of)＋数词表示，常用的表达有：

总数为 a total of　　　　　　连续数为 a series of

为期 a period of　　　　　　最大值为 a maximum of

最小值为 a minimum of　　　发生率为 an incidence of

死亡率为 a mortality of　　　精确率为 an accuracy of

平均数为 an average of/a mean of   平均持续时间为 an average duration of

随访平均间隔时间为 a median follow-up interval of

例9 在住院第二天持续发热最高达 40℃。

Daily fever persisted with temperatures reaching a maximum of 40 degrees Celsius on the second hospital day.

例10 有8例院内感染,死亡率为50%。

Nosocomial infection was noted in 5 patients with a mortality of 60%.

如果一连串的名词各附有不同数值,就不宜采用以上结构。可用"名词,数值"的表示法。

例11 被抗体包裹的细菌与临床综合征的关系是:无症状细菌尿15%;膀胱炎8%;急性出血性膀胱炎67%;前列腺炎67%;急性肾盂肾炎62%。

The relationship of antibody-coated bacteria to clinical syndromes was: asymptomatic bacteriuria, 15%; cystitis, 8%; acute hemorrhagic cystitis, 67%; prostatitis, 67%; and acute pyelonephritis, 62%.

Task 11 **Translate the following sentences into English.**

1. 我们对56名80岁老人进行了体检。

_____

2. 肺癌的总死亡率降低了50%。

_____

3. 只要经常锻炼并养成良好的饮食习惯,你的新陈代谢就会增加10%。

_____

4. 30%的癌症患者可以用此化验检测,假阳性误差率不到5%。

_____

5. 头2例患者在夜间住院,故未做血糖分析。这就使患者分别延迟16及12小时才进行适当的治疗。

_____

Glossary

A

admonition /ˌædməˈnɪʃən/ n. 警告，劝告

afferent /ˈæfərənt/ adj. 传入的

alveolar /ælˈviːələ/ adj. (alveoli n.,
  pl. alveolus) 肺泡的

amelioration /əˌmiːljəˈreɪʃən/ n. 改善，改良，改进

amino /ˈæmɪnəʊ/ adj. 氨基的

analogy /əˈnælədʒi/ n. 类比，比拟

antagonism /ænˈtæɡənɪzəm/ n. 对抗，对立，拮抗

antigen /ˈæntɪdʒən/ n. 抗原

antioxidant /ˌæntiˈɒksɪdənt/ n. 抗氧化剂

aorta /eɪˈɔːtə/ n. (pl. aortae/aortas) 主动脉

apex /ˈeɪpeks/ n. (pl. apices /ˈeɪpɪˌsiːz/) 顶尖

appendectomy /ˌæpənˈdektəmi/ n. 阑尾切除术

appendicitis /əˌpendɪˈsaɪtɪs/ n. 阑尾炎

arcuate /ˈɑːkjʊɪt/ artery /ˈɑːtəri/ 弓状动脉

arsenical /ɑːˈsenɪkəl/ adj. 砷的

arteriole /ɑːˈtɪəriəʊl/ n. 小动脉

asthma /ˈæsmə/ n. 哮喘

atelectasis /ˌætəˈlektəsɪs/ n. 肺不张

atheroma /ˌæθəˈrəʊmə/ n. (pl. atheromas,
  atheromata) 粥样斑

atherosclerosis /ˌæθərəʊsklɪəˈrəʊsɪs/ n. 动脉粥样
  硬化

atrium /ˈeɪtriəm/ n. 心房

atropine /ˈætrəʊpiːn/ n. 阿托品

B

barrier /ˈbæriə/ n. 障碍物，屏障

bereft /bɪˈreft/ adj. 丧失……的；被剥夺……的

beneficence /bɪˈnefɪsəns/ n. 仁慈，善行

benzonatate /benˈzəʊnə/ n. 苯佐那酯

bolster /ˈbəʊlstə/ v. 支持

bronchial /ˈbrɒŋkiəl/ adj. 支气管的

C

calyx /ˈkeɪlɪks/ n. (pl. calyces) 盏

capillary /kəˈpɪləri/ n. 毛细血管

carcinoma /ˌkɑːsɪˈnəʊmə/ n. (pl. carcinomas,
  carcinomata) 癌

causation /kɔːˈzeɪʃən/ n. 因果关系

cellular /ˈseljʊlə/ adj. 细胞的，细胞质的；细胞
  状的

cervix /ˈsɜːvɪks/ n. 颈部，子宫颈

chemoprophylaxis /ˌkeməʊˌprɒfiˈlæksɪs/ n. 化学
  预防，化学品预防

chemoreceptor /ˈkeməʊrɪseptə/ n. 化学受体，化
  学感应器

cholera /ˈkɒlərə/ n. 霍乱

chromosome /ˈkrəʊməsəʊm/ n. 染色体

coagulable /kəʊˈæɡjʊləbl/ adj. 可凝结的

collagen /ˈkɒlədʒən/ n. 胶原质

colon /ˈkəʊlən/ n. 结肠

commission /kəˈmɪʃən/ n. 委托，委任

complementarity /ˌkɒmplɪmenˈtærɪti/ n. 补充，互
  补性

complicate /ˈkɒmplɪkeɪt/ v. 并发疾病

complication /ˌkɒmplɪˈkeɪʃən/ n. 并发症

condom /ˈkɒndəm/ n. 避孕套，安全套

congenital /kɒnˈdʒenɪtl/ adj. (指疾病等)生来的，
  先天的

constipation /ˌkɒnstɪˈpeɪʃən/ n. 便秘

contractile /kənˈtræktaɪl/ adj. 可收缩的，有收缩
  性的

coronal /ˈkɒrənl/ adj. 冠状的

cortex /ˈkɔːteks/ n. (pl. cortices /ˈkɔːtɪsiːz/ or
  cortexes)皮质

corticomedullary junction 皮髓质结合

curare /kjʊˈrɑːri/ n. 箭毒

cystic /ˈsɪstɪk/ adj. 胞囊的；膀胱的；胆囊的

cytokine /'saɪtəʊkaɪn/ *n.* 细胞因子

cytopathology /ˌsaɪtəʊpəˈθɒlədʒi/ *n.* 细胞病理学

D

degeneration /dɪˌdʒenəˈreɪʃ(ə)n/ *n.* 退化；变性

demographic /diːməˈɡræfɪk/ *adj.* 人口统计学的

dendritic /denˈdrɪtɪk/ *adj.* 树枝状的

denervate /diːˈnɜːveɪt/ *v.* 除神经支配，去神经

dextromethorphan /ˌdekstrəʊmiːˈθɔːfən/ *n.* 右美沙芬

determinant /dɪˈtɜːmɪnənt/ *n.* 决定因素

diabetes /ˌdaɪəˈbiːtiːz/ mellitus /məˈlaɪtəs/ 糖尿病

dismutase /dɪsˈmjuːteɪs/ *n.* 歧化酶

diverticular /ˌdaɪvəˈtɪkjʊlə/ *adj.* 憩室的，膨部的

dose-dependent *adj.* 取决于剂量的

E

elastin /ɪˈlæstɪn/ *n.* 弹性蛋白

elucidate /ɪˈluːsɪdeɪt/ *v.* 阐明，说明

embryo /ˈembriəʊ/ *n.* 胚胎

emesis /ˈeməsɪs/ *n.* 呕吐

empathic /emˈpæθɪk/ *adj.* 移情作用的，感情移入的，共情的

encode /ɪnˈkəʊd/ *vt.* 编码

endogenous /enˈdɒdʒənəs/ *adj.* 内生的，内源的

enzyme /ˈenzaɪm/ *n.* 酶

eosinophilia /ˌiːəˌsɪnəˈfɪliə/ *n.* 嗜曙红细胞过多，嗜曙红细胞增多

epidemiology /ˌepɪˌdiːmiˈɒlədʒi/ *n.* 传染病学，流行病学

ethical /ˈeθɪkəl/ *adj.* 伦理的，道德的

evanesent /ˌevəˈnesənt/ *adj.* 逐渐消失的

exogenous /ekˈsɒdʒənəs/ *adj.* 外生的，外源的，由外生长的

exquisite /ɪkˈskwɪzɪt/ *adj.* 精致的；强烈的

extracellular /ˌekstrəˈseljʊlə/ *adj.* （位于或发生于）细胞外的

F

familial /fəˈmɪliəl/ *adj.* 家族的，家族遗传的

fibrosis /faɪˈbrəʊsɪs/ *n.* 纤维症

forensic /fəˈrensɪk/ *adj.* 法医的，应用法律程序的

G

gamut /ˈɡæmət/ *n.* 全域，全范围

geriatrics /ˌdʒeriˈætrɪks/ *n.* （作单数用）老年病学

glomerular /ɡlɒˈmeruːlə/ *adj.* 肾小球的

glomerulus /ɡlɒˈmeruːləs/ *n.* （*pl.* glomeruli /ɡlɒˈmeruːlaɪ/）（肾）小球

glottic /ˈɡlɒtɪk/ *adj.* 声门的

glucose /ˈɡluːkəʊs/ *n.* 葡萄糖

H

haematology /ˌhiːməˈtɒlədʒi/ *n.* 血液学，血液病学

hagfish /ˈhæɡfɪʃ/ *n.* 蒲氏黏盲鳗

hemophilia /ˌhiːməʊˈfɪliə/ *n.* 血友病

herbicide /ˈhɜːbɪsaɪd/ *n.* 除草剂

hilum /ˈhaɪləm/ *n.* （*pl.* hila）门

histopathology /ˌhɪstəʊpəˈθɒlədʒi/ *n.* 组织病理学

homeostasis /ˌhəʊmiəʊˈsteɪsɪs/ *n.* 稳态，内稳态

homeostatic /ˌhəʊmiəʊˈstætɪk/ *adj.* 稳态的

hybrid /ˈhaɪbrɪd/ *n.* 混合体，混合物

I

idiopathic /ˌɪdiəˈpæθɪk/ *adj.* 自发的，特发的

immunization /ˌɪmjuːnaɪˈzeɪʃən/ *n.* 免疫

immunodeficiency /ˌɪmjuːnəʊdɪˈfɪʃənsi/ *n.* ［生］免疫缺陷

incision /ɪnˈsɪʒən/ *n.* 切口

indication /ˌɪndɪˈkeɪʃən/ *n.* 指征，适应证

infarction /ɪnˈfɑːkʃən/ *n.* 梗死

infestation /ˌɪnfeˈsteɪʃn/ *n.* 侵染

inflammation /ˌɪnfləˈmeɪʃən/ *n.* 红肿，炎症

inguinal hernia /ˈɪŋɡwɪnəl/ /ˈhɜːniə/ 腹股沟疝

inhibitor /ɪnˈhɪbɪtə/ *n.* 抑制剂

innate immunity 固有免疫

innervate /ɪˈnɜːveɪt/ *vt.* 分布神经，刺激

in situ /ɪn ˈsaɪtjuː/ *adj.* 原位的

intercostal /ˌɪntə(ː)ˈkɒstl/ *adj.* 肋间的

intrinsically /ɪnˈtrɪnsɪkəli/ *adv.* 内在地；固有地，实质地

intussusception /ˌɪntəsəˈsepʃən/ *n.* 肠套叠

irrigate /ˈɪrɪɡeɪt/ *vt.* 冲洗

L

lamprey /ˈlæmpri/ *n.* 八目鳗，七鳃鳗

laparoscopy /ˌlæpə'rɒskəpi/ *n*. 腹腔镜检查

leucine /'ljuːsiːn/ *n*. 亮氨酸，白氨酸

lymphocyte /'lɪmfəsaɪt/ *n*. 淋巴细胞

M

macromolecule /ˌmækrəʊ'mɒləkjuːl/ *n*. 大分子，高分子

magnitude /'mægnɪtjuːd/ *n*. 大小；规模；数量

mastectomy /mæs'tektəmi/ *n*. 乳房切除术

metabolism /mə'tæbəlɪzəm/ *n*. 新陈代谢

microbe /'maɪkrəʊb/ *n*. 微生物

milieu /mɪ'ljuː/ *n*. 环境

mitosis /mɪ'təʊsɪs/ *n*. （细胞的）有丝分裂

modification /ˌmɒdɪfɪ'keɪʃən/ *n*. 修改，修正

morphology /mɔː'fɒlədʒi/ *n*. 形态学

mortality /mɔː'tælɪti/ *n*. 死亡率

myalgia /maɪ'ældʒiə/ *n*. 肌痛

myocardial /ˌmaɪəʊ'kɑːdiəl/ *adj*. [解]心肌的

N

narcotic /nɑː'kɒtɪk/ *adj*. 麻醉的，镇静的

navel /'neɪvəl/ *n*. 脐

nephron /'nefrɒn/ *n*. 肾单位

neutrophil /'njuːtrəfɪl/ *n*. 嗜中性粒细胞

non-insulin-dependent *adj*. 非胰岛素依赖型的

O

off-label /'ɒf ˌleɪbl/ *adj*. 超说明书用药的，未经临床试验认可的

osteoporosis /ˌɒstɪəʊpə'rəʊsɪs/ *n*. 骨质疏松症

outmoded /aʊt'məʊdɪd/ *adj*. 过时的

P

Papanicolaou /ˌpæpəˌnɪkəʊ'leɪuː/ 帕帕尼古拉乌（希腊医师和解剖学家）

papilla /pə'pɪlə/ *n*. (*pl*. papillae /pə'pɪliː/) 乳突

paralyze /'pærəlaɪz/ *vt*. 使……瘫痪

parasite /'pærəsaɪt/ *n*. 寄生虫

parenchyma /pə'reŋkɪmə/ *n*. 实质

pathology /pə'θɒlədʒi/ *n*. 病理学，病理；病状

perforation /ˌpɜːfə'reɪ(e)n/ *n*. 穿孔

periphery /pə'rɪfəri/ *n*. 外周，周围

peritonitis /ˌperɪtəʊ'naɪtɪs/ *n*. 腹膜炎

pertussis /pə'tʌsɪs/ *n*. 百日咳

pesticide /'pestɪsaɪd/ *n*. 杀虫剂

pertinent /'pɜːtɪnənt/ *adj*. 相关的

phagocytic /ˌfægəʊ'sɪtɪk/ *adj*. 噬菌细胞的，吞噬细胞的

pharmacological /ˌfɑːməkə'lɒdʒɪkəl/ *adj*. 药物学的，药理学的

pharmacology /ˌfɑːmə'kɒlədʒi/ *n*. 药物学，药理学

pilocarpine /ˌpaɪlə'kɑːpiːn/ *n*. 匹鲁卡品，毛果芸香碱

polymath /'pɒlɪmæθ/ *n*. 博学的人

postulate /'pɒstjʊleɪt/ *vt*. 要求，假定

potent /'pəʊtnt/ *adj*. 强有力的，有效的

profile /'prəʊfaɪl/ *n*. 侧面，轮廓；图表，图谱

predispose /ˌpriːdɪ'spəʊz/ *v*. 易患某病，易感

pus /pʌs/ *n*. 脓

R

radical /'rædɪkəl/ *n*. [化]基

ramification /ˌræmɪfɪ'keɪʃən/ *n*. 分叉，分支；衍生物

randomly /'rændəmli/ *adv*. 任意地，随机地

receptor /rɪ'septə/ *n*. 感受器，受体

rectal /'rektəl/ *adj*. 直肠的

reinforce /ˌriːɪn'fɔːs/ *vt*. 加固，加强，增强

renal /'riːnl/ *adj*. 肾的

renal pelvis /'pelvɪs/ 肾盂

replicate /'replɪkeɪt/ *v*. 复制

residuum /rɪ'zɪdjʊəm/ *n*. 残余，剩余

retard /rɪ'tɑːd/ *n*. 迟延，减速

retroperitoneal /ˌretrəʊˌperɪtə'nɪəl/ space 腹膜后隙

rupture /'rʌptʃə/ *n*. & *v*. 破裂

S

schizophrenia /ˌskɪzəʊ'friːniə/ *n*. 精神分裂症

selenium /sə'liːniəm/ *n*. 硒

sequela /sɪ'kwiːlə/ *n*. (*pl*. sequelae) 后遗症

shunt /ʃʌnt/ *n*. 分流管

sickle-cell anemia 镰状细胞血症

spectrum /'spektrəm/ *n*. 系列，范围；光谱

sputum /'spjuːtəm/ *n*. 痰

superoxide /ˌsjuːpə'rɒksaɪd/ *n*. 过氧化物

susceptible /səˈseptəbl/ adj. 易受外界影响的，易受感染的

syncope /ˈsɪŋkəpi/ n. 晕厥

synonymous /sɪˈnɒnɪməs/ adj. 同义的

syphilis /ˈsɪfɪlɪs/ n. 梅毒

systemic /sɪsˈtemɪk/ adj. 全身的

T

tailor /ˈteɪlə/ vt. 调整，使适合

telltale /ˈtelteɪl/ adj. 泄露内情的，报警的

tendon /ˈtendn/ n. ［解］腱

tertiary /ˈtɜːʃəri/ adj. 第三的，第三位的

thebesian /θiːˈbiːziən/ veins 心最小静脉（特贝西乌斯静脉）

theorem /ˈθɪərəm/ n. 定理

three-dimensional /ˌθriːdaɪˈmenʃənəl/ adj. 三维的

thoracic /θɔːˈræsɪk/ adj. 胸的，胸廓的

toxicology /ˌtɒksɪˈkɒlədʒi/ n. 毒理学，毒物学

transcription /trænsˈkrɪpʃən/ n. ［生物学］转录，信使核糖核酸的形成

trypanosome /ˈtrɪpənəˌsəum/ n. 锥体虫

tuberculin /tjuːˈbɜːkjuːlɪn/ n. 结核菌素

tuberculosis /tjuːˌbɜːkjuˈləusɪs/ n. 肺结核

tumor /ˈtjuːmə/ n. 肿块，肿瘤

tussive /ˈtʌsɪv/ adj. 咳嗽的

U

undergird /ˌʌndəˈgɜːd/ vt. 从底层加固，加强

ureter /juəˈriːtə/ n. 输尿管

urinalysis /ˌjuːrɪˈnælɪsɪs/ n. 尿液分析

V

vaccine /ˈvæksiːn/ n. 疫苗

vanilloid /vəˈnɪlɒɪd/ n. 香草酸

vascular /ˈvæskjələ/ adj. 血管的，脉管的

ventricle /ˈventrɪkl/ n. （脑、心）室

vertebra /ˈvɜːtɪbrə/ n. 脊椎骨，椎骨